		Effects on the Skin
VITAMIN D (calciferol; cholecalciferol)	Milk, cod liver oil, butter, wheat cereals, bananas.	Facilitates healing of scars. Contributes to the formation of the bones.
VITAMIN E (alpha-tocopherol)	Milk, butter, veal liver, wheat cereals, bananas.	Has a toning effect on the muscles and a firming effect on the skin.
VITAMIN H (biotin)	Wheat cereal, oatmeal, beans, peas, liver, kidney.	Very important to the skin. Helps prevent scaling dermatitis and the skin from becoming a greyish color.
VITAMIN PP (nicotinamide; niacin)	Milk, egg, cereals, oatmeal, liver, yeast, kidney, pork, rice.	Prevents pellagra. Helps prevent hypersensitivity (small pimples) to the sun.
PROTEIN	Milk, cheese, yogurt, wheat cereals, oatmeal, beans, lentils, beef, pork, lamb, veal, chicken, turkey, goose, duck, sole, haddock, perch, cod, shrimp, tuna fish, salmon.	Contributes to the formation of tissues, muscles, hair, and nails. Helps repair and replace tissues. Is a great source of energy.
CALCIUM	Milk, cheese, yogurt, broccoli, oranges, almonds, salmon, sardines.	Contributes to the formation of bones and teeth. Helps blood coagulate. Aids growth in childhood.
IRON	Cereals, lima beans, lentils, almonds, liver, heart, beef, turkey, oysters.	Carries oxygen in the blood and contributes to the formation of the red corpuscles.

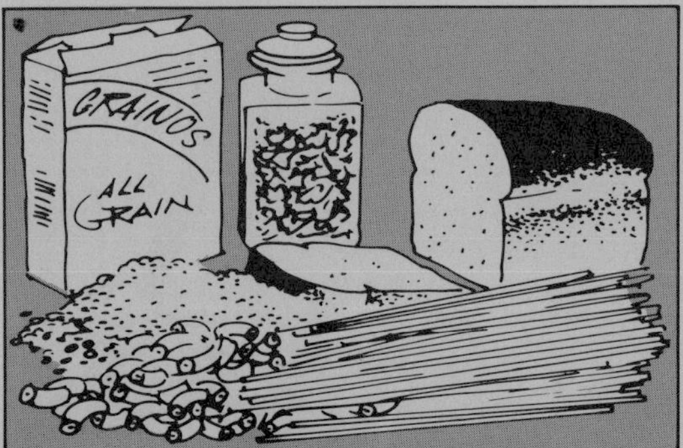

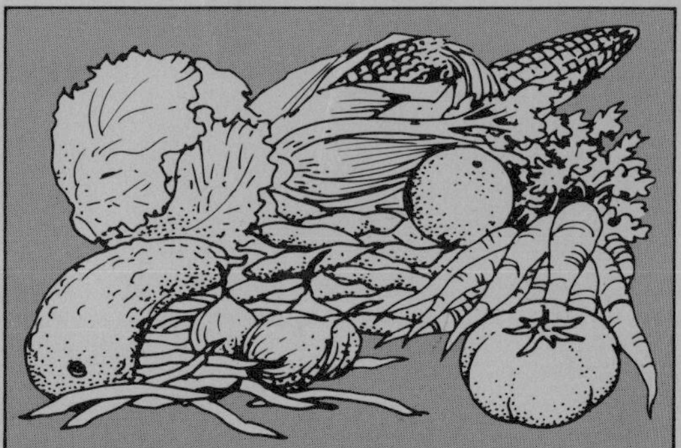

The Professional Skin Care Manual

Prentice-Hall, Inc., *Englewood Cliffs, New Jersey 07632*

SUZANNE TREMBLAY

Esthetics Consultant

The Professional Skin Care Manual

Library of Congress Cataloging in Publication Data

TREMBLAY, SUZANNE (date)
The professional skin care manual.

Bibliography: p:
Includes index.
1. Beauty culture. 2. Skin—Care and hygiene.
I. Title.
TT958.T73 642.7'26 78-4167
ISBN 0-13-725358-3

The Professional Skin Care Manual
Suzanne Tremblay

Printed in the United States of America

10 9 8 7 6 5 4 3 2 1

PRENTICE-HALL INTERNATIONAL, INC., *London*
PRENTICE-HALL OF AUSTRALIA PTY. LIMITED, *Sydney*
PRENTICE-HALL OF CANADA, LTD., *Toronto*
PRENTICE-HALL OF INDIA PRIVATE LIMITED, *New Delhi*
PRENTICE-HALL OF JAPAN, INC., *Tokyo*
PRENTICE-HALL OF SOUTHEAST ASIA PTE. LTD., *Singapore*
WHITEHALL BOOKS LIMITED, *Wellington, New Zealand*

Contents

Foreword

Esthetics is, by definition, the science of beauty, and an esthetician is a person who has received training in skin care and hygiene. An esthetician also employs special techniques and products to preserve the skin's suppleness and elasticity and to keep it healthy and looking young.

In writing this book, Suzanne Tremblay, an esthetician, teacher, consultant, and administrator in the cosmetic industry, has provided estheticians with an indispensable tool. The book was written with the awareness of a current pressing need for effective training in the practice of esthetics. From an immense amount of scientific information available, Mrs. Tremblay has extracted the essential principles and the practical and theoretical developments needed by the esthetician in her practice.

This book will be of tremendous value, for without claiming to be a substitute for the classical books on esthetics, it answers a definite need and closes the existing gap between the theory and practice of esthetics.

Thus, we are grateful to the author who, through her expertise in all areas of esthetics, was able to select and describe in understandable language, the material that will be of the greatest value to professional estheticians and to anyone interested in this science.

Denise Gillet Robert
Consultant
Esthetics and Cosmetology

Introduction

Femininity and the desire to look young and attractive are reasons why esthetics has enjoyed such growth in the last few years. Yet, in order to trace the origin of the use of perfumes and cosmetics, we must go back into history and even into prehistoric times.

In the beginning, perfumes and powders were kept only for religious ceremonies. Later, the use of perfume became commercialized, first in Egypt and then in Greece and Rome, and thus was no longer considered sacred. The Egyptians were really the first people to develop the use of cosmetics for purposes of beautification. Cosmetics became widely used, largely because of the influence of Cleopatra, the Queen of Egypt. But technical progress was very slow. Makeup, in particular, was always made from a base of lanolin, olive oil and, especially, pork lard. During the seventeenth and eighteenth centuries, most cosmetics were produced in home industries and sold in only a few rare shops.

It was not until the nineteenth century, with the advent of modern chemistry, that the cosmetic industry really began to flourish, primarily because of the availability of almost limitless possibilities of new excipients. As a result, there was an abundance of new products, equipment, and beautification techniques that opened the way to a new profession—*esthetics.*

Today, even after several years of progress, research, and discoveries within the profession, it is still very difficult to find practical texts needed to teach esthetics. At the urging of departments of specialized education in both Canada and the United States, and at the request of several manufacturers of products and equipment, I decided to collect all the relevant and necessary information into a single volume. My objective was, precisely, to provide estheticians, cosmetologists, students, and anyone else interested in skin care with a simplified text containing all the information needed to teach or practice esthetics.

Keeping the skin healthy must be the primary goal of the esthetician and thus, she must fully understand the skin's composition and functions. For this reason, the early chapters of this book are devoted to the study of the cell, the skin, and some of the tissues connected to the skin.

Other subjects included are pH, personal and professional hygiene, psychology, skin analysis, various cleansing techniques, massage, and makeup. There is a discussion of different kinds of electrical equipment—their application and directions for use. Skin changes, various products used in esthetics—their classification and composition—and the kinds of treatment that are useful for different skin types are also described.

Montreal, Quebec SUZANNE TREMBLAY

The Professional Skin Care Manual

1

The Cell

For decades, makeup has been used to conceal certain imperfections in the skin. It has been known for some time, however, that makeup does not always hide imperfections but sometimes accentuates them. Thus, we now realize that it is important to treat the inside of the skin by adopting healthy nutritional habits and a good diet recommended by a physician. The outer portion of the skin can be treated through a program of daily cleansing, moisturizing, and regular care in collaboration with an esthetician.

DEFINITION

It is important, therefore, for the esthetician to study the cell, for it is the smallest particle of living matter and the basic component of every part of the human body: the organs, tissues, glands, muscles, and so forth, are composed of small juxtaposed cells, which reproduce themselves by constant division.

The skin is composed of a multitude of cells, which divide and reproduce in the basal or germinative cell layer of the skin and eventually die in the horny layer.

The esthetician must always remember that healthy skin renews itself constantly and regularly every three to four weeks. Thus, she must nourish the cell source, and to do that, she must know the ways in which the skin can be penetrated.

The skin is crisscrossed by its own system of glands that is somewhat unequally distributed. There are sudoriparous glands, which secrete sweat and moisturize the skin, and sebaceous glands, which secrete sebum. The latter soften the skin and lubricate the hair by keeping an oily film on the surface, thus preventing the epidermis from drying out.

The most important thing for the esthetician to know is that, because of the skin's impermeability, the only means of penetrating it to nourish the basal cell layer is through the sebaceous gland canal, called the *ostium.* This is the only opening by which a product can penetrate into the skin. Thus, the esthetician must study all the aspects of the skin, starting with the cell, the tissues, muscles, and so forth, in order to understand the principles behind each treatment and how to obtain the maximum benefit for clients.

Definition: The cell is the smallest particle of living matter that, when totally isolated, can survive and reproduce.

Cell Structure: Cells are composed of two essential portions, the cytoplasm and the nucleus.

Cytoplasm: Cytoplasm is a viscous, transparent gellike substance. It is living material that moves with so-called cytoplasmic motion. It contains, among other things, various constituents called enclaves or reservoirs.

Cell Membrane: The cell membrane is a thin, flexible, permeable film or skin that surrounds the cytoplasm. Because of its permeability, the membrane permits cellular exchange for nourishment and life support of the cell. The cell membrane is composed of proteins and lipids.

Inert Components

Vacuoles: Vacuoles are cavities that contain an aqueous fluid (waste material evacuated by the cell).

Enclaves or Reservoirs: The enclaves are small droplets of lipids or glucides, which are diffused throughout the cytoplasm. They are produced by the cell to store food to meet the needs of the organism.

Living Components

Mitochondria: The mitochondria furnish the necessary energy to the cell for its growth, reproduction, and other vital functions.

Endoplasmic Reticulum:	The site of protein and enzyme synthesis.
Golgi's Apparatus:	Golgi's apparatus comprises a network of very fine fibers extended between the cells that appear to be involved in the functions of secretion and excretion.
Lysozymes:	The lysozymes are the cell components that contain digestive enzymes.
Centrosome:	The centrosome exists as a nodule located near the nucleus. It plays a very important part in cell division.
The Nucleus:	The nucleus is the essential part of the cell. It is composed of a viscous, granular (nuclear) substance of greater consistency than that of the cytoplasm. The nucleus is contained within a very thin nuclear membrane. The nucleus comprises approximately one third to one quarter of the cell. If the nucleus becomes too large, the cell may die.
Nucleoles:	Nucleoles are spherical bodies, surrounded by the chromatin network.
Chromatin:	Chromatin is a granular, irregular substance which is transformed into chromosomes during cell division.

The chromosomes appear at the moment of cell division. They are the small filaments that carry the genes, the latter being responsible for hereditary traits (qualities, defects, and illnesses that are inherited).

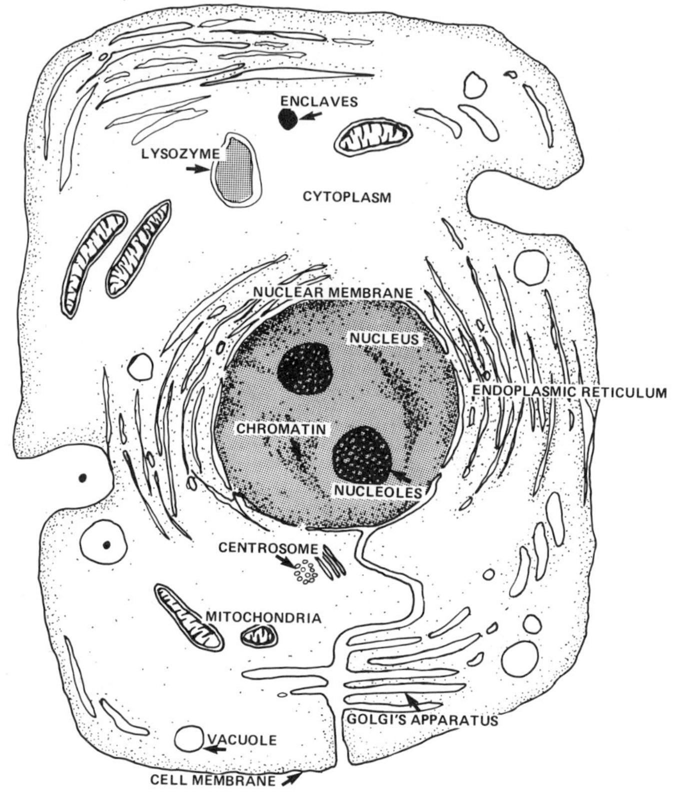

The cell

THE FUNCTIONS OF THE CELL

Manifestations of Cell Life

Sensitivity. Cells react to all impulses in a specific manner depending on their location in the organism or the cellular group to which they belong. For example, the cells which form the muscles (muscle cells) contract when a nervous stimulation is applied, whereas after heat stimulation, cells of the sudoriparous (sweat) glands react by secreting perspiration.

Nourishment. The cell draws its nourishment from the blood plasma, which contains all the indispensable elements of its survival: organic substances, minerals, and water. Nutrients are absorbed by the cell in the aqueous state and are able to enter the cytoplasm through the membrane because of the latter's selective permeability. The membrane lets only useful substances penetrate into the cytoplasm and allows harmful substances to be excreted. Food crosses the membrane by a physical phenomenon known as osmosis. Thus, a cell is nourished and survives by the processes of absorption and excretion.

Metabolism. Metabolism is a term denoting all the transformations that occur in a living organism, including anabolism and catabolism.

Anabolism. Anabolism is the transformation of nutritive substances into living tissues (assimilation phase).

Catabolism. Catabolism is the transformation of materials absorbed by the tissues into energy (dissimilation phase).

Respiration. A cell breathes by drawing in oxygen (usually dissolved in water) from the environment outside its wall.

Growth. The cell grows because of the absorbed nutrients which are generally transformed into energy or new tissue. When the cell reaches its maximum size, it stops growing in order to form another cell.

Cellular Division

Multiplication. Certain cells, such as the white blood cells, multiply by direct division, also known as amitosis. In this process, the cytoplasm and nucleus become drawn out and divide directly into two parts.

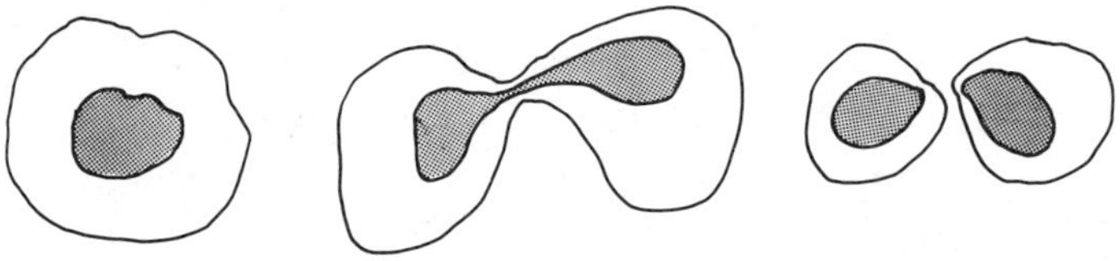

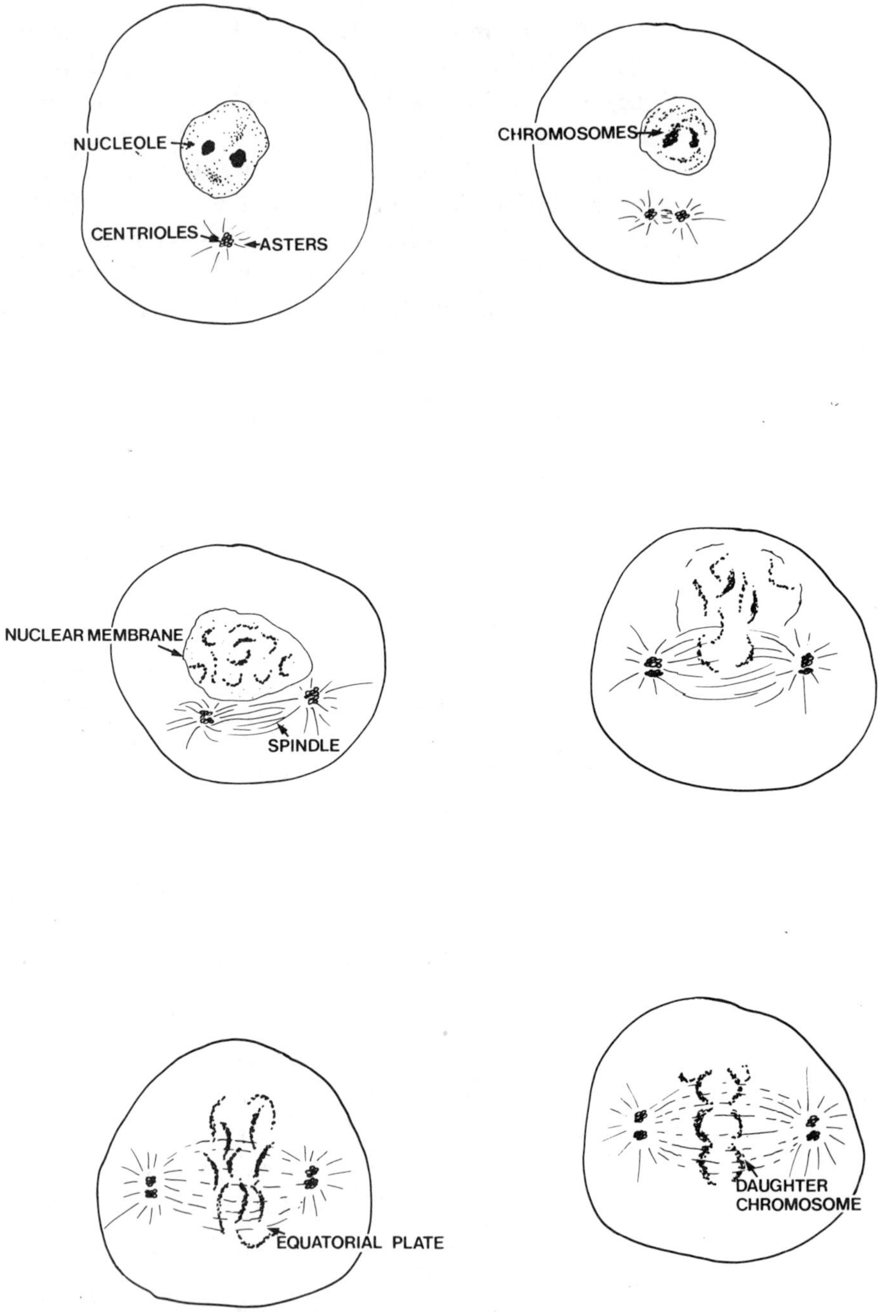

Stages of mitosis

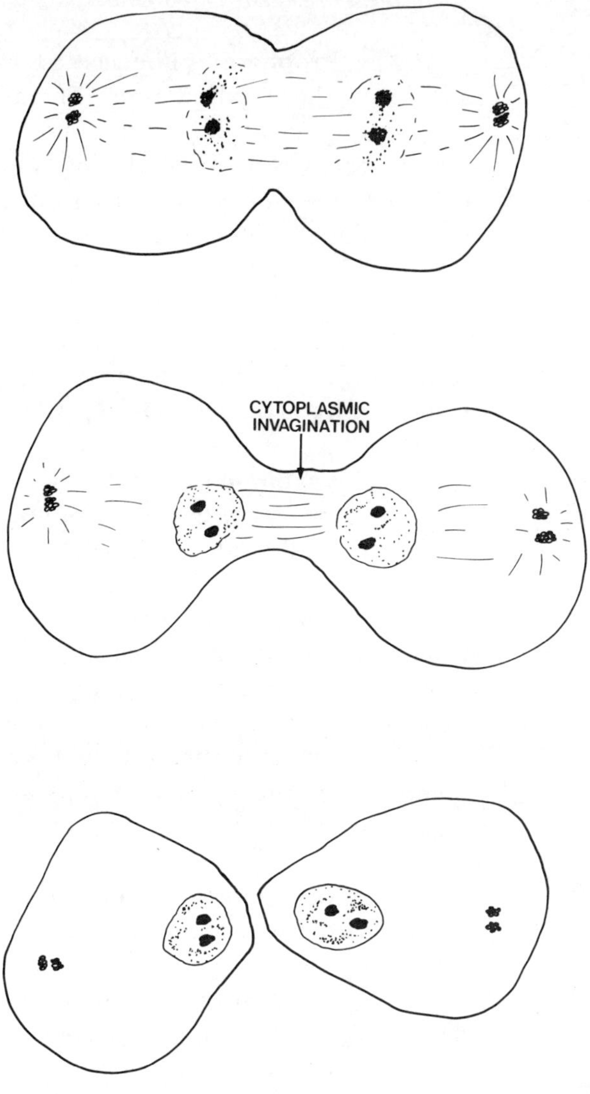

Stages of mitosis (*continued*)

Indirect Division or Mitosis. The majority of cells multiply by indirect division. Indirect division or mitosis in a multicellular animal, such as man, is totally different from amitosis and involves several phases as outlined on the next page.

The Prophase. The centrosome is enclosed by filaments and forms the so-called aster. The aster divides in two, and each portion migrates toward the opposite poles of the cell while still joined together by a spindle of filaments. The nucleus becomes enlarged; the nucleoles and chromatin reorganize and form the chromosomes. The chromosomes then divide lengthwise and thicken. The nuclear membrane disappears.

The Metaphase. The chromosomes shift toward the equator of the cell. The two asters are visible at the two poles of the spindle. This is the *equatorial plate.*

The Anaphase. The divided chromosomes separate to form two identical daughter chromosomes. These chromosomes move along the spindle toward the asters.

The Telophase. The filaments of the asters become less distinct and the daughter chromosomes continue their outward movement. The nucleoles reappear. At each pole of the cell, two new nuclei are visible. The dividing cell then becomes drawn in at the center, and the cell membrane is invaginated in such a manner that the cytoplasm separates, yielding two cells. Thus when the cell division is complete, two new cells are formed.

The Interphase. The cell ceases all reproductive activity and prepares for another division.

The duration of cellular division varies from 30 minutes to 3 hours, depending on the type of cell.

THE TISSUES

The skin is composed of different layers of tissues, each having specific functions and properties. The esthetician must study each of these carefully in order to provide effective treatment for the clientele.

The epithelium, with its packed structure, plays a protective role, for it is in contact with the environment. Connective tissue, because of its elasticity and toughness, carries out a supportive function and connects all the tissues and organs to one another. Finally, there are very specific tissues, such as the blood tissue, which distributes the necessary nutrients for life support via a system of blood vessels; the lymph tissue, which collects wastes and helps form scar tissue over wounds with its white cells; nerve tissue; and so forth.

The term *tissue* is applied to a group of like cells, which are connected and carry out identical functions. There are two major categories of tissues: supporting tissues (connective tissue for example) and specialized tissues (blood, nerve, muscle, lung, and other tissues).

The Epithelium

All tissues (or organs) are also protected by an epithelium (the outer protective tissue), which is the portion coming into direct contact with the outside or any free surface of the organism. The skin, for example, has an epithelium, which is the outermost portion in contact with the environment. Lungs also possess an epithelium, which comes in contact with the thoracic cavity. There are two main categories of epithelium: simple and stratified.

Simple Epithelium: Formed from a single layer of cells.

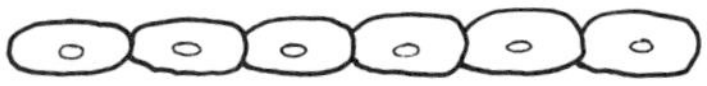

Stratified Epithelium: Composed of several rows of overlapping cells. The cells can all be the

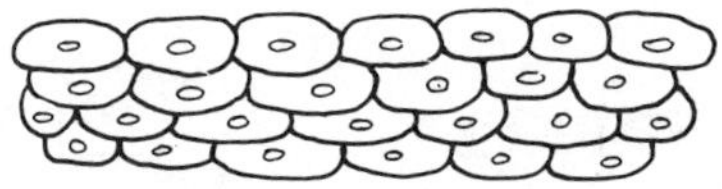

same or can vary from one layer to another. Thus, it is the superficial layer that serves as the epithelium.

In each of these two categories, depending on the organ or tissue to be covered, the epithelium can take on different forms.

Cubical: Cells which are as wide as they are long.

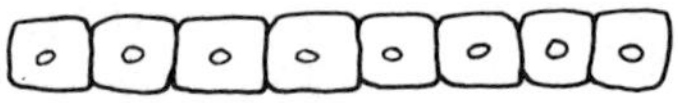

Simple Cubical Epithelium. Example: the epithelium protecting the surface of the ovary.

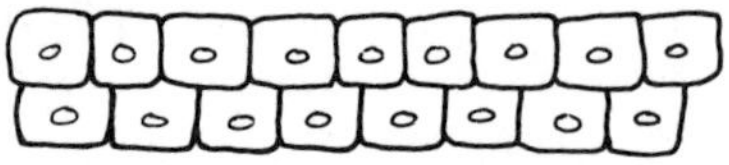

Stratified Cubical Epithelium. Rather rare and usually formed of only two layers of cells. Example: excretory canals of the sweat glands.

Pavement: Composed of flat cells resembling bricks or tiles, which are much longer than they are wide.

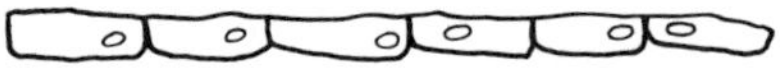

Simple Pavement Epithelium. Example: the cells that cover the pulmonary alveoli.

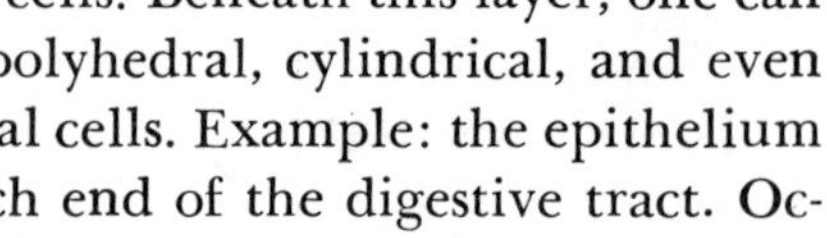

Stratified Pavement Epithelium. The superficial layer is composed of pavement cells. Beneath this layer, one can find polyhedral, cylindrical, and even cubical cells. Example: the epithelium at each end of the digestive tract. Occasionally, this stratified pavement epithelium is keratinized or horny. In this state, several layers of hardened cells, forming what is called the horn, can be found on the side closest to the exterior. Example: the epithelium covering the skin.

Cylindrical: The cells are cylindrical in form, being much higher than they are wide.

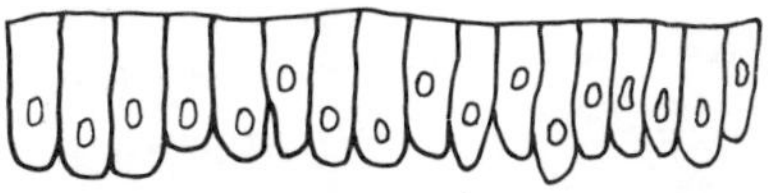

Simple Cylindrical Epithelium. Example: the epithelium covering the middle portion of the digestive tract.

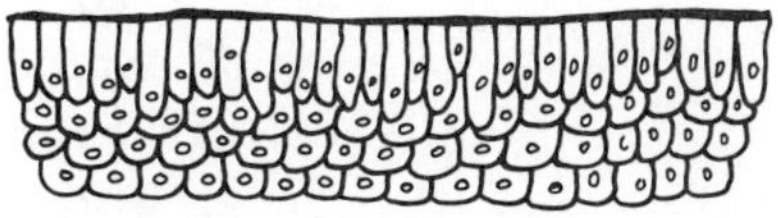

Stratified Cylindrical Epithelium. The superficial layer of this epithelium is cylindrical, whereas the other layers are formed of larger or smaller polyhedral cells. Very rare. Example: a certain region of the ureter.

Role of the Epithelium. Because of its packed cellular structure, the major function of the epithelium is to protect the underlying tissues from external influences. It is an actual barrier, obstructing contaminants from the outside. In addition, the epithelium serves as a medium of exchange with the environment, being involved in absorption, excretion, and secretion processes. The epithelium can also be regarded as the receptor site of external stimulations (e.g., touch).

Certain epithelial tissues possessing specialized structures (vibratile cilia or muscle fibers) also perform a motor function. For example, the bronchial epithelium pushes mucus toward the mouth via its vibratile cilia.

Supporting, or Connective Tissues

Unlike epithelial tissue, connective tissue is composed of cells that are separated from one another and diffused throughout an abundant intercellular material called "ground substance." Depending on the type of tissue, the consistency of the ground substance varies, but it always contains clusters of fibrous collagen. (See illustration on bottom of page 15.)

Collagen is a protein, rich in glycocoll (aminoacetic acid). Collagen is insoluble in water, but when it is heated in water, it turns into a soluble gelatin substance (used in the preparation of certain glues).

The Fibrous Connective Cell. The fibrous connective cell, also called a fibroblast, possesses an irregular shape, usually with an elongated spindle resembling fine branching filaments. This cell is responsible for the formation of both fibrillar material and the ground substance.

Reticular Tissue. Besides the components just described, connective tissue contains reticular fibers. The number of fibers depends on the type of tissue it is. Reticular fibers are much finer than collagen fibers and tend to form supportive networks for certain organs. They exist in large numbers in the connective tissue of the spleen and in bone marrow.

Elastic Tissue. Elastic connective tissue fibers can be characterized as stretchable and very strong. They can exist as isolated fibers or as clusters which actually form an elastic strip (ligaments). Elastic tissue is very common in subcutaneous tissue.

Types of Connective Tissue

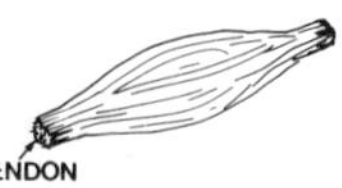
TENDON

Fibrous Tissue. This type of connective tissue is noted for its resistance to rupture. It is essentially comprised of solid and nonstretchable collagen fibers. It forms the tendons and ligaments.

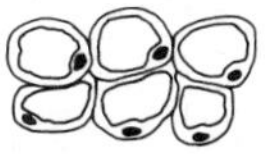

Adipose Tissue. These tissue cells are made up of lipids (fat). The cytoplasm is reduced to a thin border. Adipose cells can be found as single cells or in small clusters, or they can be isolated in the connective tissue. When they become very numerous and predominate over other cells, they form adipose tissue.

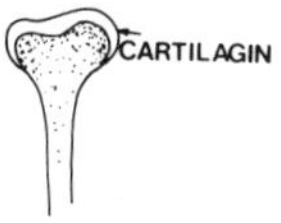

Cartilaginous Tissue. Solidified connective tissue formed principally of a substance called cartilagin. This tissue is found in the joints.

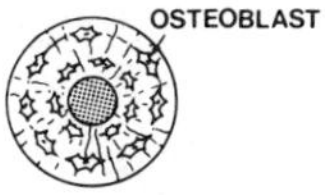

Bony Tissue. Connective tissue whose basic material is impregnated with calcium salts which gives it its characteristic rigidity. Star-shaped bone cells are called osteoblasts.

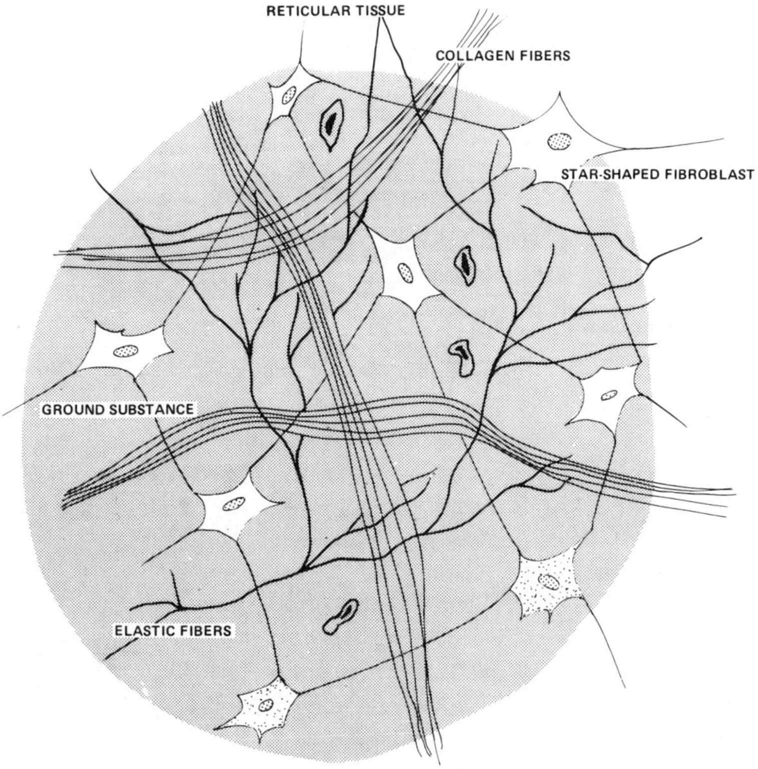

Connective tissue

Functions of Connective Tissues

As the name implies, connective tissues support, protect, and join other tissues or organs together. The bony and cartilaginous tissues provide particularly rigid support. Because they are strong, elastic, and tear-resistant, connective tissues also play a mechanical role. One of the special characteristics of some connective tissues is their ability to change forms during the development of the organism. In other words, one type of cell can be transformed directly into another type—a process known as *metaplasia.*

Specialized Tissues

Blood Tissue. In humans and in all other vertebrates, the blood is a red, viscous liquid. It circulates in the vascular system and is distributed to all the organs in order to carry the necessary nourishment for life. The normal pH of blood in man ranges from 7.3 to 7.4.

Blood is composed of red cells (erythrocytes) and white cells (leukocytes), which are suspended in the plasma.

Erythrocytes. These cells (red blood cells) contain hemoglobin, which gives the red color. The hemoglobin traps oxygen and carbon dioxide and transports both substances throughout the human body.

Leukocytes. These cells (white blood cells; phagocytes) are colorless cells found throughout the body. They absorb and thereby eliminate any deal cells, bacteria, or foreign bodies that have accidentally been introduced into the body. Leukocytes fight off foreign microbes by forming antibodies whenever there is a wound or infection.

Plasma. Plasma is the liquid portion of blood. Its function is to receive substances for assimilation (constructive metabolic products) . Plasma comprises 55 percent of the blood and contains mineral salts, proteins, glucides, lipids, and water.

The Lymph. The lymph is a clear, yellowish liquid that contains white blood cells, mostly lymphocytes. The lymph circulates very slowly throughout the intercellular spaces and in a special vascular system of lymphatic vessels. The lymph constantly bathes the cells of the organism, assists in cell nourishment, and collects waste material for elimination. The white cells within the lymph also help in the process of scar formation over a lesion. Lymph is a far less rich fluid than blood but is more abundant. It is able to traverse the walls of the blood vessels, move toward the blood, and then return.

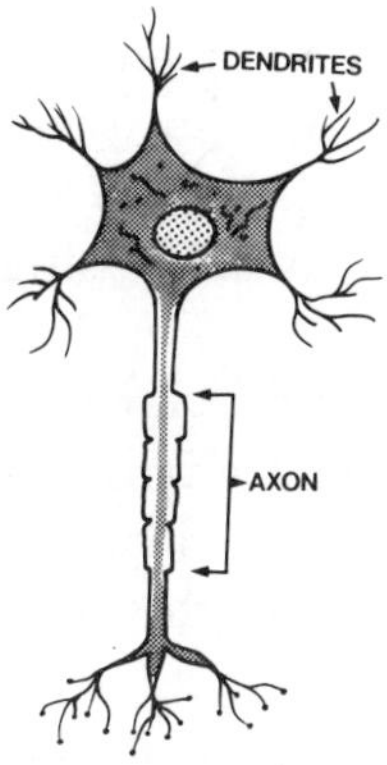

Nervous Tissue. This tissue acts as a conductor. It is the basic component of the brain, the spinal marrow (in the vertabrae), and the nerves which join the organs of the nervous system to all other parts of the body. Nerve cells, or neurons, possess long fibers that conduct nervous impulses from other organs or from outside the organism. There are two types of nerve fibers. *Dendrites:* conduct nervous impulses toward the cells from other organs or from outside the body. *Axon:* the single central core of a neuron, which conveys impulses from the neuron to other cells.

Muscular Tissue. Tissues formed from elongated cells called muscular fibers, which allow the muscles to contract. One may distinguish between two main categories of muscular fibers: smooth fibers and striated fibers.

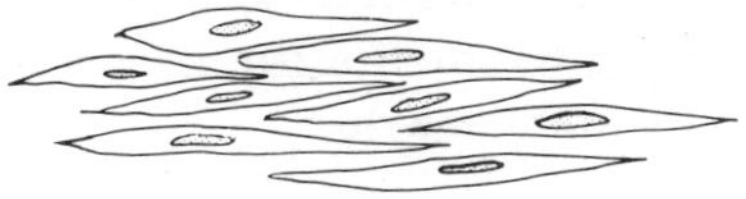

Smooth fibers: Constitute the smooth muscular layers of the viscera (stomach, intestines, bladder) and the vessels of the circulatory system. The smooth muscles are involved in the involuntary movements of all the so-called "hollow" organs (except the heart), causing them to perform the motions of relaxation and contraction.

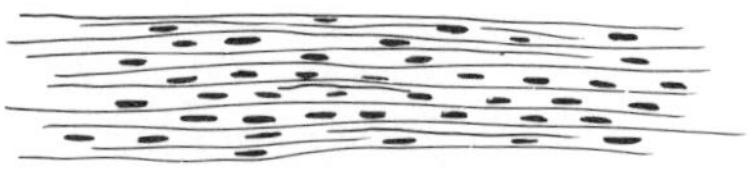

Striated fibers: In contrast to the smooth fibers, these fibers contract voluntarily. They constitute the skeletal muscles, forming the fleshy portions of the body.

THE MUSCLES

The esthetician's concern is always to give treatment that will provide the clients with the best results. To accomplish this, a thorough knowledge of the muscles, their direction, and elasticity is necessary, for their overrelaxation is responsible for wrinkles and sagging in the skin. It is of the utmost importance that the esthetician understand the musculature of the face, neck, and décolleté before starting any skin treatment because all cleansing, massage, and application of creams, masks, serums, and so forth, must always follow the direction of the muscle fibers. Muscles are the organs of movement. They are characterized as possessing elasticity and contractility.

Since this book will discuss esthetic massage, particularly of the face, neck, and décolleté, it is necessary to be perfectly familiar with the muscles in these areas and their functions. It is of the utmost importance that the massage movements follow in the same direction as the muscle fibers.

All the muscles of the neck and head are quite delicate because they possess very fine fibers. They easily become slack, not only with time but also following psychological stress or frequent overly vigorous massages. Such factors lead to muscle sagging, including flabbiness of the skin and premature wrinkling. Therefore, movements for face and neck massages must be performed extremely gently.

Functions of the Major Muscles of the Face and Neck

Forehead or Frontal Muscle:	Controls the movement or creasing of the forehead. When it contracts, it shifts the skin of the scalp and determines the formation of the transverse wrinkles of the forehead.
Orbicular Muscle of the Eyelid:	Controls the movements of the eyelid and is involved in the formation of vertical wrinkles around the eyelid (the crow's-feet).

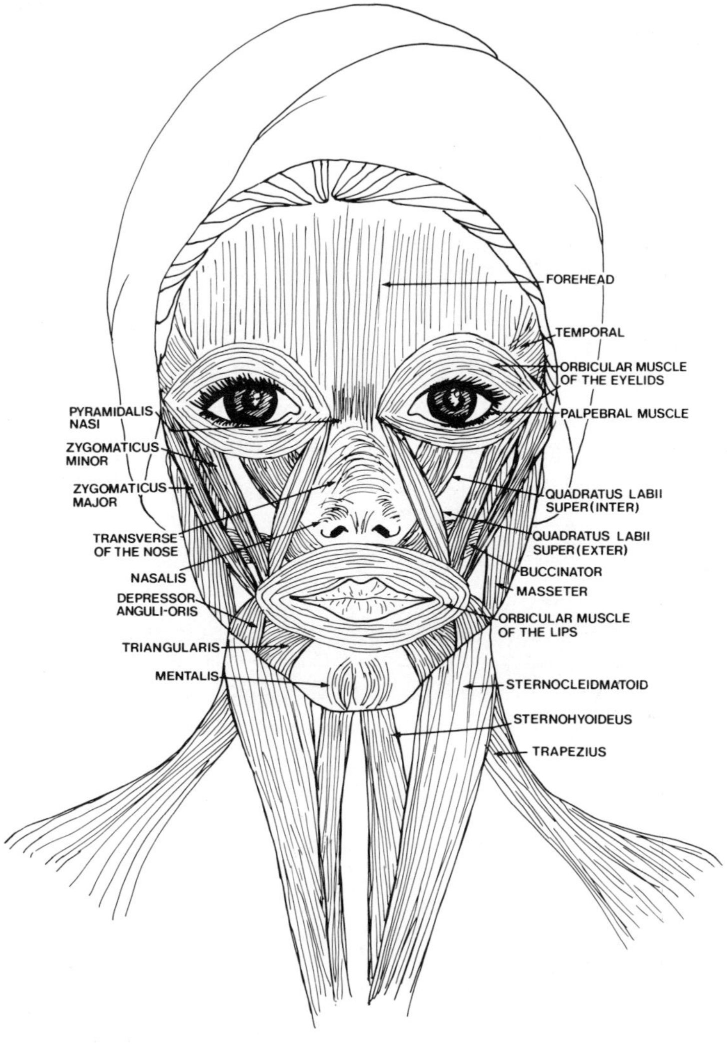

Principal muscles of the head and neck

Orbicular Muscle of the Lips:	Controls the movements of the lips. When this muscle contracts, the lips either compress inward or protrude outward.
Masseter and Temporal Muscles:	Both muscles are involved in the chewing process. The masseter raises the mandible while the temporal closes the mouth and causes the jaw to move forward and to the side.
Sternocleidomastoid Muscle:	Flexes the spinal column to enable the head to bow and controls the rotation of the head.
Trapezius Muscle:	Contributes to the movements of the shoulders and arms and is the muscle with which one pulls one's head back.

2

The Skin

Since the esthetician's primary objective is to keep the skin healthy, it is unthinkable for her not to possess a complete knowledge of the skin's structure, its vascularization, functions, and chemical composition. She must therefore pay particular attention to this chapter because in it are found the fundamentals of all types of treatment.

In this chapter and the one following, the esthetician will learn the difference between a sudoriparous gland (which secretes sweat and whose tubular shape prevents products from penetrating into the skin) and a sebaceous gland (which possesses an opening called an *ostium,* the only means of penetration to the basal cell layer of the skin where mitosis takes place). The exterior appearance of the skin depends entirely on the activity within the basal cell layer.

DEFINITION

The skin forms the protective covering over the entire surface of the body. The color of the skin varies according to race, individual variation, the season, location on the body, and age. When examined by the naked eye, the surface of the skin shows deep hollows formed when the joints or muscles contract. In older persons, lines on the skin deepen around the face (the mouth, eyes, and forehead), forming wrinkles or deep furrows, which result from skin flaccidity and dehydration.

Shallow grooves, which look like sharp pencil lines, also appear on the palms of the hands and the soles of the feet. These are papillary ridges or linear protrusions, which crisscross each other forming complex patterns. These patterns are different for each individual and even provide a means of identifying a person (fingerprints).

Examined under a magnifying glass, the skin appears to be covered by crisscrossing lines or hatchmarks, which may or may not be very prominent. The ostia, very tiny openings, are little hollow depressions through which the sebaceous glands secrete sebum. Fine hairs and barely visible pores can also be seen; the pores are the outlets for the sweat glands. It is important to distinguish between pores and ostia because the two are frequently confused.

The thickness of the skin varies from 0.2 mm to 3 mm (or from 1/50 to 1/6 in.).

STRUCTURE OF THE SKIN

The skin is primarily composed of two layers—the epidermis at the surface and the dermis underneath. The dermis is made up of connective tissue. Within it lie the true dermis and the hypodermis. The latter connects the skin to the muscles.

Epidermis

The epidermis is stratified pavement epithelium, composed of five layers of cells, the most superficial of which are keratinized. The five layers, from the innermost to the outermost layer, are called:

1. Basal cell layer (stratum germinativum)
2. Malpighi layer (stratum mucosum)
3. Langerhans layer (stratum granulosum)
4. Layer of Oehl (stratum lucidum)
5. Horny layer (stratum corneum)

The name desquamative layer is given to the cells of the horny layer, which are those that peel off (exfoliate) on the exposed side.

The Basal Cell Layer (Stratum germinativum). The basal cell layer is located on the dividing line between the dermis and the epidermis. It is composed of a single layer of cells, which constantly divide, giving birth to cells for all the other layers. Here mitosis is the most common form of cell division. Within this layer, melanin, the substance responsible for skin pigmentation, is produced. When the skin is exposed to the sun, melanin production (the process of tanning) increases.

The migration of cells from the basal cell layer to the horny layer is of extreme importance in esthetics, for it is the biological activity of the basal cell layer that gives the skin a young and healthy look.

It takes from three to four weeks for cells to migrate from the basal cell layer to the desquamative horny layer. In a young orga-

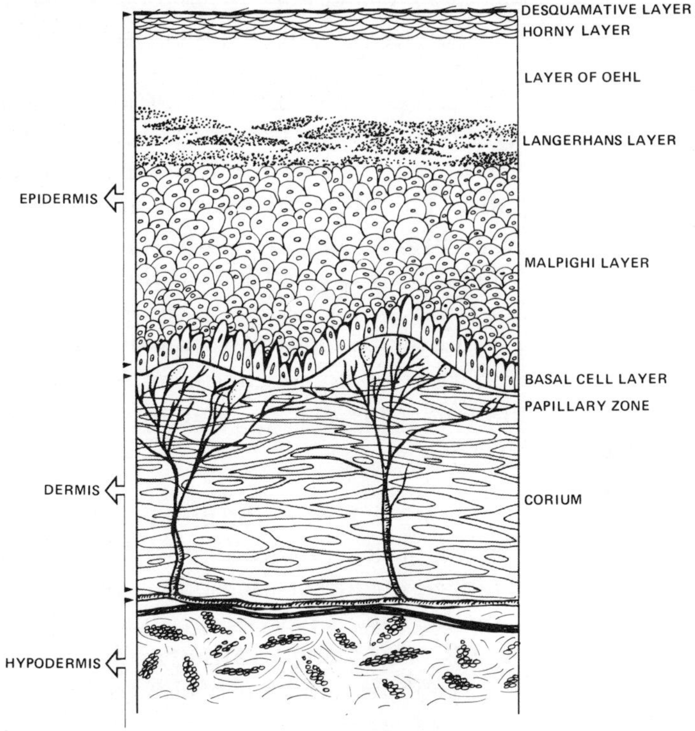

The skin

nism, the rate of metabolism is faster, and cellular waste material is eliminated regularly. The tissues therefore maintain their vitality and firmness. The metabolism slows down with age, and oxygenation of the tissues becomes less efficient; that is, waste material not eliminated by the metabolic process accumulates in the cells and actually poisons them. Thus, any nutritional problem in the cells of the basal layer induces abnormalities in their development (dehydration, keratinization, loss of elasticity, wrinkling).

Malpighi Layer (Stratum mucosum). The Malpighi layer is composed of several layers of polyhedral cells, which are fairly flat as they climb toward the next layers. The cells of the Malpighi layer are very active; the cytoplasm is more dense and filled with different substances (cholesterol, amino acids). They are joined together very closely by filaments called tonofibrils. They show what the adult form of epidermis cell looks like.

Langerhans Layer (Stratum granulosum). Langerhans layer is composed of one or several layers of flat granular cells. The egg-shaped nucleus indicates that cell death commences at this point. The tonofibrils have completely disappeared. Granules of keratohyaline appear in the cytoplasm; this is a fatty substance which permeates and softens the skin's keratin.

Layer of Oehl (Stratum lucidum). The layer of Oehl is a thin layer of homogenous, transparent cells. It is at this level of the epidermis that cellular death actually occurs and the horny layer starts.

Horny Layer (Stratum corneum). The horny layer is formed of several dead cells, 15 to 20 lamellas. These cells are arranged on top of each other like the layers of a shell, and they form keratin. They are gradually eliminated by desquamation, usually one by one (scaling) or in certain pathological conditions (e.g., sunburn) in large peeling sections.

The epidermis contains no blood vessels and only a few nerve endings. It is nourished by osmosis via the capillaries of the dermis.

The horny layer is a highly efficient protective shield. One of its most important roles is to prevent evaporation of essential moisture from the tissues. The absence of blood vessels constitutes another protective aspect of the epidermis, since the only possible areas of entry are the openings for the sebaceous glands. The structure of the latter, however, minimizes the danger of foreign organisms entering the body. In another chapter we will see how these natural obstacles to penetration can be used to advantage in esthetics.

The Dermis

The dermis is the true skin, comprising two distinct sections: the true dermis and the hypodermis. It is composed of connective tissue and contains blood and lymph vessels as well as nerve endings. (Tactile corpuscles, also called Meissner's corpuscles, are fibrous capsules containing nerve fibers sensitive to touch.) The dermis also contains glands and hair follicles. It is nourished by diffusion.

The True Dermis or Corium

Outer Layer—Papillary Zone. The papillary zone is essentially composed of loosely formed connective tissue comprising scarcely one fifth of the total thickness of the dermis. At its surface are found the dermal papillae (papillae corii), which project from the dermis to the epidermis and correspond precisely to the undulations or folds of the epidermis. The papillae, which contain the blood capillaries, are responsible for the nutrition of the epidermis.

Inner Layer—Corium. The corium or inner layer of the dermis is primarily composed of collagen fibers. It is formed of a more dense connective or supportive tissue, making up the remaining four fifths of the thickness of the dermis. Besides collagen, the inner layer contains elastic fibers (elastin), numerous blood vessels emerging from a subcutaneous vascular system, sensory nerves, which transmit impulses from the skin and lymph vessels. It is this layer which gives the skin the resistance and elasticity that permit it to resist external mechanical influences.

Hypodermis. The hypodermis is a thick region composed of loose connective tissue. It serves as a fat storage and insulating layer. The hair follicles are rooted in the hypodermis, and the principal sweat glands are also located there. (Cellulitis develops in the hypodermis.)

VASCULARIZATION OF THE SKIN

The skin is highly vascularized. Blood circulation is more concentrated in the face than in any other area of the skin. This is of great importance in esthetics. The veins and arteries form a primary network (subdermal plexus) between the dermis and hypodermis where the cells are less compressed and elongated. Vessels emerge from the subdermal plexus, traverse the dermis, and lead to a second network or plexus, located in the upper portion of the dermis just below the papillae (subpapillary plexus). This second plexus forms a capillary loop to each papilla with an ascending arterial branch and a descending venous branch. These loops are very compact. The arterioles emerge from this plexus to nourish the dermal papillae, the sweat and sebaceous glands, and the epidermis. Because the epidermis contains no capillaries, it receives nourishment from the dermis by diffusion.

The skin also contains numerous lymph vessels, the flow of which parallels the direction of arterial and venous flow. The lymph vessels originate in the papillae from which they drain the lymph vehicle for all organic wastes, to deeper levels. Any type of facial massage, the most fundamental aspect of esthetics, facilitates the drainage of the lymph and enhances arterial and venous circulation.

The Nerves and the Nervous System of the Skin

The nerve system within the skin gives rise to a multitude of different sensations: touch, thermal impulses (hot and cold), and pain. There are so many nerves in the skin that it may be thought of as a vast sprawl of nerve endings.

The free (peripheral) sensory endings can be found in great numbers at different levels of the epidermis, but always below the Langerhans layer. The majority of nerve endings are located in the dermis or hypodermis and are produced by various tactile corpuscles (the Meissner, Krause, Pacini and Ruffini corpuscles) and tactile rings. Each of these endings has a particular sensitivity (to hot, cold, pressure, and so forth).

Sensory nerves are accompanied by motor nerves, which spread to the muscles from the skin, directing those muscles that control facial expressions and those at the base of the sweat and sebaceous glands. Vasoconstrictor and vasodilator nerves envelop the blood vessels. That is why, in esthetics, the beauty of one's complexion depends not only upon cleansing the skin but also on the various methods of facial massage, effleurage, and so forth, which stimulate the nerve endings and nerves, thus increasing the blood flow. These methods can produce truly remarkable results.

GENERAL FUNCTIONS OF THE SKIN

Protection

The skin has a protective function by virtue of its ability to

Withstand physical influences: Because of its smooth, resistant, and elastic covering and its fatty hypodermic region, the skin is able to absorb external shocks and pressures.

Withstand chemicals and water: The horny cells, keratin, fatty tissues, and sebum of the skin prevent excess water, liquids, or chemicals from penetrating.

Protect against wounds and microorganisms: The skin's immediate and constant regeneration of cells and its acidic pH enable it to protect the body from wounds and microorganisms.

Protect against the sun or ultraviolet radiation: The skin affords protection from these elements with the help of the horny layer, keratin and melanin, which rise from the basal cell layer toward the upper layers and tan the skin to prevent burns. Sebum and sweat also defend the body against ultraviolet and infrared radiation.

Respiration

In man, the tissues of the skin, like all tissues, breathe. (Oxygen is absorbed and carbon dioxide is exhaled.) However, skin respiration is very weak.

Thermal Regulation

One of the most important functions of the skin is its capacity to regulate, or control, body temperature. When the body becomes overheated, that is, when the internal temperature is elevated, vasodilation occurs in the skin. This increases the volume of blood circulating (giving the skin higher color) and the amount of perspiration secreted. If the temperature is too low, vasoconstriction takes place. Then the diameter of the blood vessels decreases by contraction. Less blood is passed, skin color fades, perspiration decreases. These processes allow the body to conserve its warmth and protect itself against cold and are responsible for the skin reddening when hot and becoming white in the cold.

Secretion

External. The skin, through the secretions of the sweat glands, helps rid the organism of certain wastes. The sebaceous glands, which produce a secretion called sebum, force out harmful substances. (We will study these glands in more detail in the next chapter.)

Internal. The skin secretes enzymes, fermentation substances, hormones, and so forth, which participate in nutritional exchanges. The most important of the hormones secreted by the skin is histamine (a tissular hormone which produces allergic reactions).

Absorption

Absorption is the essential step in the nutrition process. Since the skin is impermeable, it is very important for the esthetician to learn to avoid all the obstacles to skin penetration. We will learn in a later chapter the various means available for avoiding these obstacles, such as cutaneous or transcutaneous absorption, imbibition through the horny layer, and so forth.

Regeneration

To the other functions of the skin, one may also add that of cellular regeneration, for the beauty and freshness of the skin depend essentially on the speed with which it can regenerate itself (approximately 30 days).

Regeneration takes place in the basal cell layer. All the cells in this layer divide in two: One of the two new cells remains in the same place while the second travels towards the next higher layer. Eventually, as the cell ages, it reaches the horny layer where it is eliminated by the desquamative layer.

Bactericidal Action

The skin is continuously in contact with microorganisms. Because the skin is acidic (i.e., it has a pH that varies from approximately 5.4 to 6.2), it effectively blocks most microorganisms from entering. That is why it is always very important in esthetics to respect and maintain the skin's acidic pH.

CHEMICAL COMPOSITION OF THE SKIN

The skin is composed of 70 percent water, 27 percent protides, 2 percent lipids, and 1 percent glucides.

Water:	Mineral salts: (in aqueous solution) Sulfur: (4 to 5 percent in the horny layer) chlorine, sodium, copper, magnesium, nitrogen, oxygen, hydrogen, calcium, iron. The skin contains one third of all the body's sodium chloride.
Protides:	Amino acids, tyrosine, tryptophane, crystine. Proteins: keratin, collagen, elastin.
Lipids:	Fatty acids, oleic acid. Sterol: neutral fatty substances such as cholesterol
Glucides:	Glucose: A small amount can be found in the horny layer.
Biocatalysts:	Enzymes: trypsin, tyrosinase Vitamins: A, H, B_6, B_3, C Hormones

3

Extensions of the Skin

The skin has its own glandular system, which is unevenly distributed in the epithelium. The glands are more or less specialized with regard to their location and the material that they secrete. The two main types of glands are distinguished according to the substance secreted: the sebaceous glands release sebum, and the sudoriparous glands sweat.

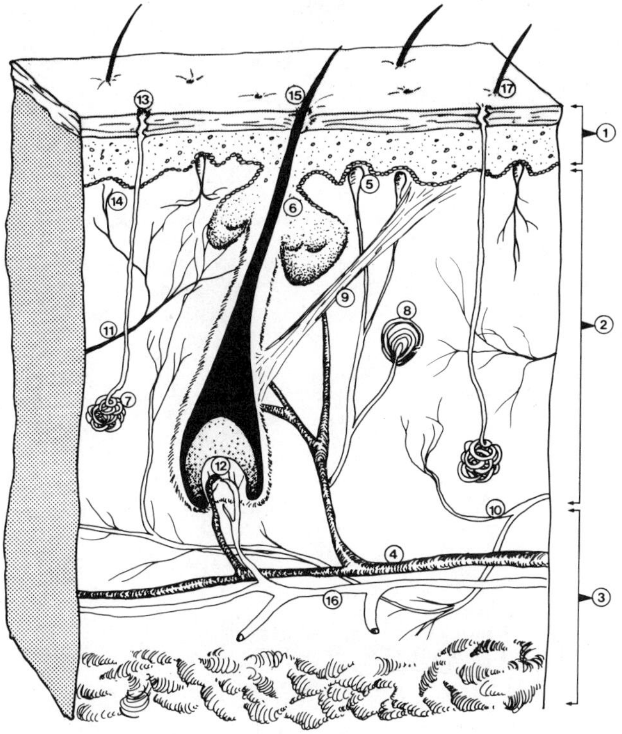

Cross section of the skin
1. artery
2. Meissner corpuscle
3. Pacini corpuscle
4. dermis
5. epidermis
6. sebaceous gland
7. sudoriparous gland
8. hypodermis
9. arrectores pilorum
10. motor nerve
11. sensory nerve
12. hair follicle papilla
13. sudoriparous gland pore
14. free sensory nerve ending
15. hair
16. vein
17. ostium

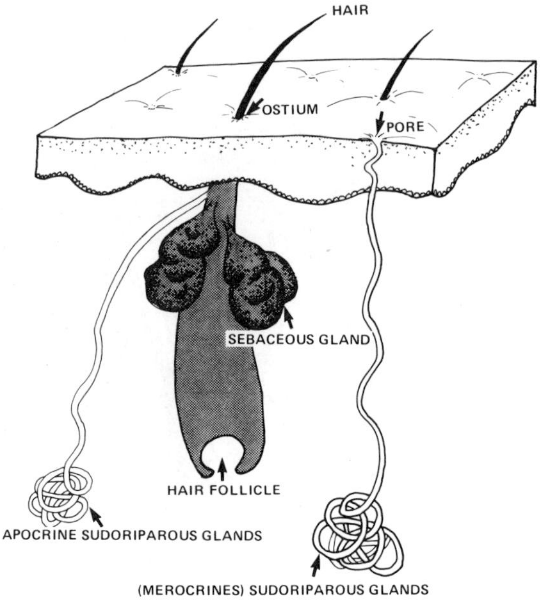

The skin glands

THE SEBACEOUS GLANDS

The sebaceous glands are small glands, found in clusters in the upper portion of the dermis. About 90 percent of them are part of the hair follicle (pilosebaceous follicle) ; a few of them open out directly onto the surface of the skin. They have different volume capacities, which are not necessarily proportionate to the size of the hair growing alongside them. The sebaceous glands are dispersed throughout the entire surface of the skin except on the palms of the hands and soles of the feet. They are particularly numerous in the scalp and face. The sebaceous glands are known as holocrine glands, that is, glands whose secreted matter (e.g., sebum) is comprised of both the entire secreting cell and its accumulated secretions. The sebum secreted by the sebaceous gland lubricates the hair and prevents the skin from drying out. Sebaceous secretions only begin at age five or six; during puberty, they increase and later maximize during young adulthood. The secretions abate in old age.

Sebum plays an important part in esthetics. When sebaceous secretions are inadequate, the epidermis becomes dry and wrinkled; when the glands secrete too heavily, the skin becomes oily and shiny. This condition of hypersecretion is known as seborrhea. Acne tends to occur in persons with seborrhea. The skin and hair constantly become very oily because sebum is continuously being regenerated regardless of the frequency of washing or shampooing.

When the sebum is blocked in the pilosebaceous follicle and unable to flow out freely, it hardens and dilates the excretory canal. The external opening then becomes plugged by cellular waste material, dirt, impurities, and so forth. This matter forms a true pimple (or comedo). Occasionally, these sebaceous accumulations enlarge and form seborrheic cysts or wens.

PILOSEBACEOUS FOLLICLE

The hair follicle represents the active portion of the hair. The first sign of the presence of a hair in humans is a thickening of the epidermis (special cell module). Such cells multiply rapidly and penetrate into the dermis from the epidermis. The follicle is thus begun from which a hair will grow.

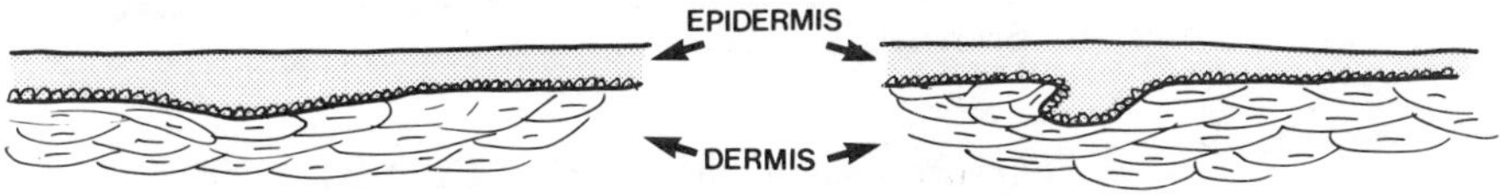

The figure illustrates the invagination of the epidermis into the dermis. The special cells continue to multiply rapidly, forming a root from which the hair will grow. Very soon, a bulbous enlargement develops at the terminal portion of this cellular thread; at its extremity, the enlarged portion invaginates to form a papilla. A sebaceous gland forms at the upper portion of the follicle, and later on in the same region, the smooth, arrector muscles of the hair appear.

The pilosebaceous follicle is composed of a short canal through which the sebum flows, as through a funnel, out to the follicle opening or ostium. From the ostium it is dispersed over the hair and surface of the skin. The ostium of the follicle, often visible to the naked eye, nearly always has a hair in the middle. The only means of penetrating the skin with a substance is through the hair follicle, thus the importance of this follicle in esthetics.

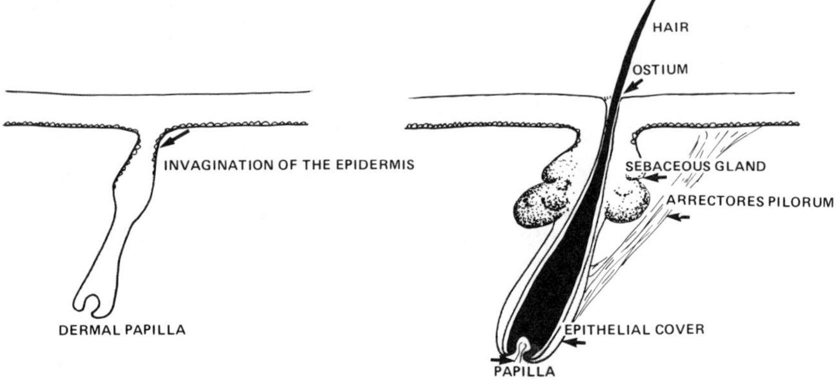

THE SUDORIPAROUS GLANDS

The sudoriparous or sweat glands are simple, tubular, convoluted glands. Some secrete as eccrine or merocrine glands, and others as apocrine glands.

Eccrine Glands (Merocrine Glands)

In humans, eccrine sudoriparous glands are the most numerous. These glands produce an aqueous secretion throughout a person's life. They are not at all related to the hair, and their only link to the epidermis is their excretory canal, which is a long tube emanating from the excretory glomerulus. The latter is located fairly deep in the dermis or occasionally in the hypodermis. The tube crosses the epidermis in a manner resembling a spiral corkscrew. In this way, it prevents dirt and foreign bodies from penetrating into it. The glomerulus is an essential part of the gland. It looks like a long, rolled-up tube and it secretes the sweat.

Sweat is composed of 95 to 97 percent water. It also contains various mineral salts, sodium chloride, some oily granulations, glucides, and waste products of cellular metabolism. The sudoriparous glands secrete sweat continuously, but the secretion is not apparent under normal conditions. When the ambient temperature increases following physical exertion or illness, there is an increase in the production of sweat. The primary function of sweat is to counteract heat, regulate body temperature, and prevent drying by hydrating the skin.

Apocrine Glands

The excretory canal of the apocrine sudoriparous glands is nearly always associated with a hair. The apocrine glands, unlike the eccrine glands, do not have a spiral-shaped canal, and for that reason they are more easily invaded by germs. They develop only at puberty and are located in regions where hair grows particularly long (the armpits, around the genital organs, and so forth).

The secretion from the apocrine sudoriparous glands has a milk-like consistency and is odorless when discharged. The odor that eventually occurs is due to surrounding bacteria. The apocrine glands are not very numerous, and they secrete only small amounts.

THE NAILS

Nails, like hair, are composed of modified skin tissue. Nails look like whitish, semitransparent plates and are located on the outermost joint of the fingers and toes.

A nail is composed of multiple layers of epithelial cells, which resemble those of all the epidermal layers except the Langerhans layer. A well-developed nail is divided into two parts. The larger part is pink in color because of the rich vascularization of the adjacent dermis below. At the base of this portion is a small, white section called the lunula. All of the nail's outward growth originates under the lunula, and the remainder of the nail simply slides passively along.

The tissue directly under the nail is called the nail bed. The cells of the basal layer proliferate and press and push other cells upward; the latter cells eventually become keratinized. The pressure exerted by the newly formed keratin forces the horny plate (the unguinal plate or nail) to slide along the nail bed to the end of the finger or toe.

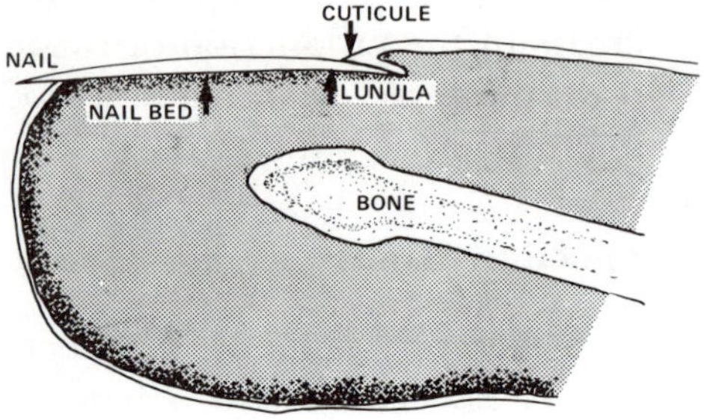

4

Means of Penetrating the Skin

In Chapter 2, we saw that the primary function of the skin is to protect, that is, to prevent moisture from escaping and foreign substances from entering the tissues. The horny layer of cells, the cutaneous fatty tissue, the sebum, and the Rein or Blank electrophysiological barrier (the different pH values in the various layers of cells in the epidermis) all help the skin perform its protective role. The outer portions of the Oehl and Langerhans layers are very acidic, while the deeper layers are less acidic or more alkaline. These differences in the pH and the resulting electrical potentials form a barrier, which gives the skin its impermeability. In esthetics, therefore, one must surmount this barrier by using one of the following methods of penetrating the skin:

1. Imbibition by the horny layer: consists of causing the outermost layer of the skin to swell temporarily.
2. Penetration through the horny layer: inducing the outer layers of skin to absorb lipid-soluble or water-soluble substances.
3. Percutaneous or transcutaneous absorption: the diffusion of a substance into the layers of the skin and possibly beyond.

IMBIBITION BY THE HORNY LAYER

Since the horny layer is composed of flat, keratinized, dehydrated, and frequently desquamated cells, it is important that it retain moisture, for moisture is the basic requirement for a beautiful complexion. To keep the horny layer moist, it is important to use high quality biological products, especially water-soluble creams (oil/water).

Method: After a light cleansing, apply a small amount of cream to the face and neck, spray a floral lotion on with an atomizer, and then massage both into the skin to enhance penetration. This causes the horney layer to swell slightly.

PENETRATION THROUGH THE HORNY LAYER

The skin prevents the evaporation of moisture everywhere except at the locations of the sweat glands. Thus the keratinized layer acts as a barrier, but with a lysing treatment or a complete cleansing, the skin becomes significantly more permeable to all lipid- and water-soluble substances. Keratin, a scleroprotein (characterized as a fibrous and insoluble body protein), allows all biological creams containing proteins, amino acids, animal oils or fats to bind themselves to it and penetrate the superficial layers of the epidermis. The horny layer subsequently swells somewhat.

> Example: an indoor tanning product (such as Quick Tanning) with a dihydroxyacetone base. Such substances combine with the keratin amino acids producing a brownish coloration, which resists washing but disappears gradually with the shedding of the cells of the horny layer.

PERCUTANEOUS OR TRANSCUTANEOUS ABSORPTION

Transcutaneous absorption is actually the diffusion of a substance into the different layers of the skin and into the circulatory and lymph systems. In esthetics we have no interest in diffusing a product into the blood or lymphatic vessels because they would then be eliminated. Our aim is to moisturize and nourish the skin in order to delay aging. It is therefore important to cross the entire thickness of the horny layer so that the active products can penetrate to the basal cell layer and to the dermis, since cellular regeneration occurs at those levels.

The only means of penetration is via the pilosebaceous follicles. Thus any substance that is able to overcome the barrier composed of sebum and cellular waste materials will likely be absorbed. The esthetician must therefore prepare the skin accordingly, namely by cleaning cellular wastes, fatty substances, sebum, and so forth, from the follicles.

> Cleansing methods: deep cleansing, cleansing with a complexion brush, gumming (refines the keratin), lysing, light peeling using enzymes (liquifies the sebum), warm vaporization (dilates the ostia), suction apparatus (draws out excess sebum from the follicles), extraction of comedones (manually or mechanically), Jacquet pinching, and so forth. After the skin is well prepared, it is important to use an active biological product, which must be lipid-soluble so that it will penetrate the skin.

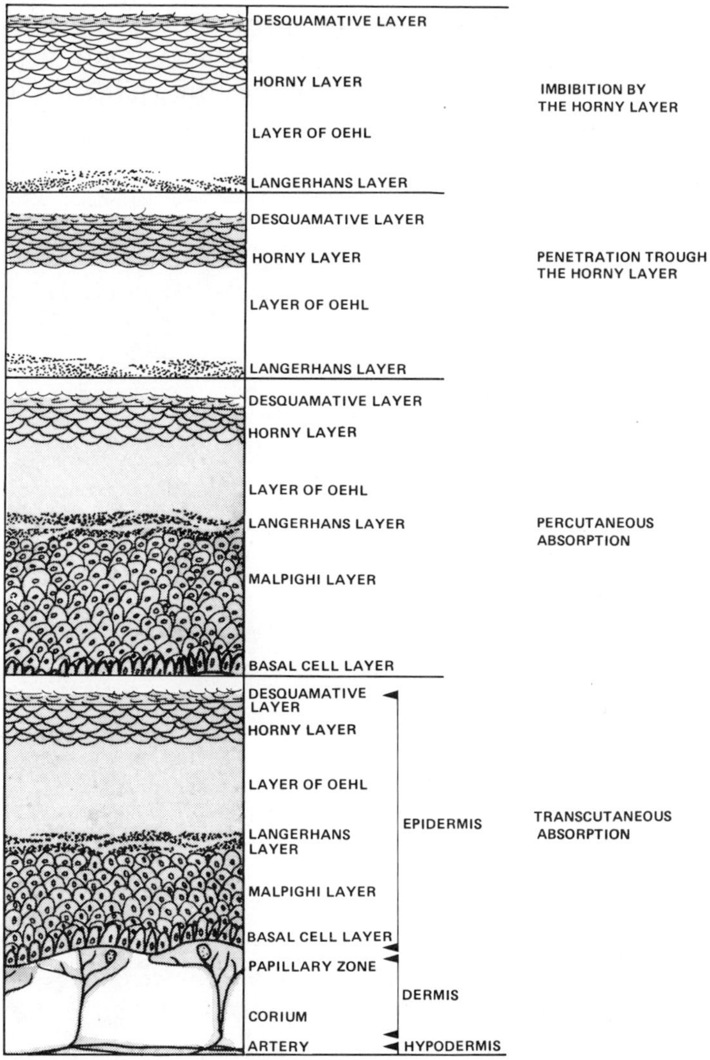

Means of penetration

The esthetician can effect penetration of a serum or active product by using manual massage, indirect massage, infrared light or galvanic current (ionization, iontophoresis) if the product is ionizable, or atomization (jet spray, hydrospray) if the product is an aqueous serum. The percutaneous route is primarily used to produce a local effect in either the epidermis, dermis, or hypodermis.

5

Classification of Skin Types

NORMAL SKIN

When speaking of normal skin, one no longer thinks, as was once the case, of a baby's skin, for one can only make a valid distinction between normal and abnormal skin after puberty.

Normal skin is smooth and velvety to the touch. It does not appear puffy or oily but resilient and firm. The pores are visible without being dilated. Normal skin does not look shiny, although the middle portion of the face is slightly more oily. It is a rosy color because of the blood actively circulating through it. It is well nourished, and the basal layer cells are rapidly regenerated. It is perfectly moisturized.

DRY OR ALIPOIDIC SKIN

Dry skin is usually rather fine and delicate but is crinkled like parchment. Underneath there is only a thin layer of oil. The pores are just barely visible. Dry skin lacks suppleness. Cellular lipids are absent, and there is insufficient secretion from the sebaceous glands.

In addition to these intrinsic factors, there are other external causes, which can dry the skin out even further. Among these we can list wind, inadequate protection, climate, overheated homes without sufficient humidification, and the use of alkaline products.

GREASY, OILY, OR SEBORRHEIC SKIN

Oily skin is usually thick and shiny. The ostia are highly visible and dilated. The levels of oil in the hypodermis are generally above normal. The grain and texture of the skin are coarse and irregular. Oily skin looks sweaty and is oily to the touch. The causes of oily skin are usually intrinsic, and it is helpful to recognize oily skin early and to start treatment before blackheads, seborrhea, or acne develop.

AGED SKIN

Aging of the skin depends not only on the person's age but also on one's state of health. Wrinkles can be prevented or delayed when you take good care of yourself and your skin. Occasionally a young person will have skin that is prematurely aged or an older person will have young, well-preserved skin.

Aging of the skin is produced by three factors: cellular intoxication, dehydration of the cells, and poor blood circulation.

Cellular Intoxication

Normal skin eliminates its cellular waste in a methodical way; however, if there is a slowdown in tissue exchange and oxygenation, the cells become intoxicated.

Dehydration of the Cells

The skin is composed of approximately 70 percent water, and if it is properly irrigated, it remains well moisturized. Tissue aging is always accompanied by drying or dehydration. As the years go by, the skin is less and less able to withstand environmental influences, illness, and so forth. Eventually it begins to degenerate, losing much of its water and being transformed into a more dense colloidal substance at every cellular level. When the skin loses its moisture, the deeper layers tend to dissipate while the upper layers, which are only slightly hydrated under normal conditions, become more dense. This is what produces keratinization.

Poor Blood Circulation

If blood circulation is poor, oxygen becomes less available for cell nourishment. A poorly vascularized organ is destined to age prematurely. In the dermis and hypodermis, collagen and elastic fibers become frayed, the dermal papillae (papillae corii) become flattened, the layer of Malpighi is regenerated more slowly, and cells accumulate at the outer layers, since they are not eliminated regularly. These extra cells make the skin appear rough, coarse, and dull.

The loss of elasticity and the reduction in the muscle mass lead to a loss of tonus and vitality. These factors provoke the deterioration of the face as a whole, and the lines of the face deepen and become more pronounced, forming wrinkles. It should be pointed out, however, that there are certain young people who have wrinkles but whose skin is still firm. These wrinkles are the lines of expression, such as the laugh lines of the face.

CHANGES IN THE SKIN

As we remarked at the beginning of this chapter it is possible to draw a valid distinction among different skin types only after

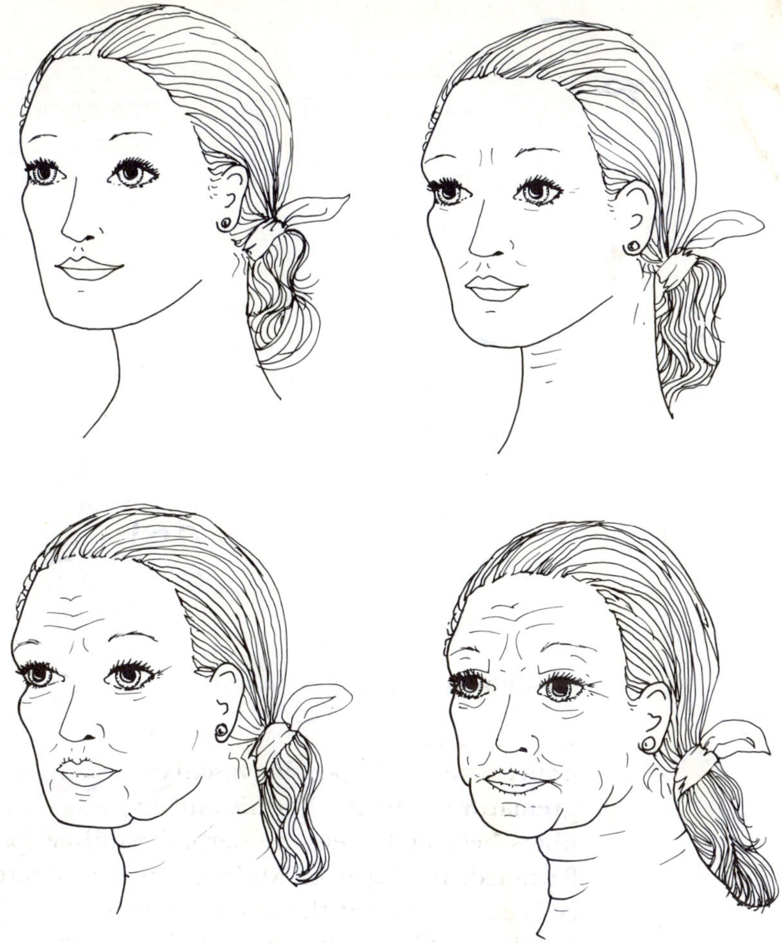

How the face ages

puberty. The changes that determine the different types of skin may be temporary or permanent.

Temporary Changes

Temporary changes usually recede spontaneously, or if they are produced by certain external factors, they can be corrected with the help of an esthetician and appropriate products. Among the most common temporary changes are

Alterations in the pH of the skin during the menstrual period or during pregnancy (the skin becomes slightly alkaline and more oily).

Peeling, dryness, dehydration due to atmospheric conditions (sun, cold) or to alkaline substances such as detergents, etc.

Permanent Changes

Permanent changes, on the other hand, are generally produced by endogenous or internal influences. When these changes persist, the skin type becomes established. Different types of alterations can actually be found on the same face. The skin types formed by permanent changes include

Coarse Skin:	When levels of oil are higher than normal in the hypodermis.
Dry or Alipoidic Skin:	When sebum secretions are insufficient.
Superficially Dehydrated Skin:	When the skin fails to retain moisture adequately and dries at the surface (desquamates).
Oily or Seborrheic Skin:	When excessive amounts of sebum are excreted.
Blotchy Skin or Erythrosis:	When the capillaries are fragile and tend to rupture or dilate.
Aged Skin:	When the connective collagen or elastic fibers harden or break and hatchmarks, wrinkles, and streaks appear.
Hyperkeratinized Skin:	When the horny layer thickens as a result of dehydration, excessive production of horny lamellae, or poor elimination of these lamellae.
Acneic Skin:	When sebum production and elimination are abnormal.

Normal skin can be kept healthy through proper care. Different types of skin can be improved by continuous appropriate treatment both at the institute and at home or, in very serious conditions, with the collaborative efforts of a physician and an esthetician.

6

The Study of pH

DEFINITION

For several years we have been hearing much about pH. Manufacturers of cosmetics do research in order to discover and make available products whose pH best suits the skin and hair.

It is important for the esthetician to know that a healthy skin must have a pH of between 5.2 and 6. She must therefore select products that will help bring the skin to its normal pH.

Before using a product in a treatment or recommending it to a client, the esthetician must measure its pH with an indicator paper or liquid. Only then can she be certain of the product's pH value and its potential effectiveness as a treatment method.

The pH is the measure of the concentration of hydrogen ions in a solution. The symbol pH is used in everyday language, and its value represents the degree of acidity or alkalinity of a substance. When a solution is neither alkaline nor acidic, it is called neutral. For example, the pH of pure water, a neutral substance, is 7. If the pH of a solution is less than 7, it is acidic; if it is greater than 7, it is alkaline.

1	ACIDIC	7	ALKALINE	14
		NEUTRAL		

Acidic:	An acidic substance is characterized by a sour taste, such as the citric acid in a lemon.
Alkaline:	An alkaline substance is the opposite of an acidic one. It has a bitter taste and shares the same properties as alkalis, such as soda, potash, ammonia.
Neutral:	A neutral substance is neither acidic nor alkaline. It falls within the intermediate area between acidity and alkalinity.

To determine whether a substance (such as a lotion, cream, milk) is acidic, alkaline, or neutral, a chemist must measure the pH or the concentration of hydrogen ions present.

The pH is used in many disciplines: in biology, in the food and dairy industries, in agriculture, and in the area that interests us—the cosmetics industry.

In biology, all vital processes are executed within a narrow pH range. With rare exceptions, life processes cannot function when the pH is less than 4.2 or greater than 8.5. The pH of a product or of the skin can be measured in two ways: electronically or colorimetrically.

MEASUREMENT OF pH

Electrometric Measurement

A pH meter is an apparatus that may be quite expensive, but that measures the pH very precisely. It is usually used in laboratories where a high degree of precision is demanded.

Colorimetric Measurement

The method used most frequently in esthetics is indicator pH paper with a range of 1 to 14. Indicator pens and solutions are also available. When dipped into a solution and then allowed to dry, indicator pH paper can give a rapid, though approximate, measure of the pH of a product when its color is compared with that of a color standard. An esthetician must always have pH papers in her possession in order to measure the pH of products before using or recommending them.

It would be desirable for the esthetician to measure the pH of her client's skin before beginning treatment or recommending a particular product. However, the pH of the skin is very difficult to measure because it is influenced by many kinds of external and internal factors that alter the pH from one day to the next or even from one hour to the next. Thus, it is not possible to give a person's exact skin pH if only one measurement is taken under only one set of conditions. The pH of the skin varies according to one's lifestyle, food, drinking habits, medications taken, soaps or cosmetics used, and so forth.

We saw in Chapter 4 that the pH of the skin is not the same in the different layers. This is the phenomenon that has come to be known as the "electrophysiological barrier" of Rein or Blank. Different pH values throughout the epidermis form electrical potentials. The pH of the horny layer of healthy skin is in the range of 5.2 to 6. In the deeper layers, it is closer to that of blood, that is, slightly less acidic or more alkaline. Blood has a pH of approximately 7.4. The pH of the epidermis is between 4.8 and 5. The esthetician therefore proceeds under the assumption that normal skin is totally acidic.

Acidic protection is provided to the skin by the fatty acids of sebum and sweat, the keratin amino acids, and by the Rein or Blank barrier. This is what we call in esthetics, the lipoprotein complex. It is absolutely necessary to maintain the skin's acidity because microbes develop more readily in an alkaline medium.

BUFFERING

The preceding paragraphs have shown that the pH provides a convenient numerical means of evaluating the acidity or alkalinity of a substance such as the skin.

Buffering is a necessary characteristic of normal healthy skin. It refers to the skin's capacity of regaining its natural acidity more or less rapidly when the normal pH balance has been disturbed by the use of alkaline substances. This natural reaction clearly demonstrates the necessity of maintaining the epidermis at its normal pH and, subsequently, the importance of using products that do not threaten the acidity of the skin.

Alkaline soaps and detergents destroy the lipoprotein complex. When this happens, the buffering mechanism starts to work. Alkali is neutralized by natural secretions and metabolic substances, which contribute to the formation of the horny layer. It takes the buffering process about three to four hours to restore the initial pH to the skin.

It is important to keep the cells of the skin from overproducing in an effort to regain normal acid levels. Such an effort results in fatigue and premature aging. Cell overproduction also activates oily secretions in skin that is already oily or greasy. Moreover, in buffering, cell production is not rapid enough and the skin remains alkaline long enough to invite microbial proliferation.

For all these reasons, the esthetician must select wisely from among all the available products while monitoring the pH in order not to disturb the acid balance of the skin.

7

Preparing for Treatment

PERSONAL HYGIENE

It is of the utmost importance that the esthetician always be neat and clean. The work area must be well organized and clean, and uniforms should be spotless. Hair should be clean and combed; long hair should be tied back. Light makeup is appropriate, but jewelry should not be worn. Fingernails should be short, clean, and well manicured; polish should not be worn because the client may have an allergy to it.

An esthetician must not forget that she is working in the regions of the face. Because of her close proximity to the client, the esthetician must be as clean and attractive as possible. (Discreet perfume, mouth wash, deodorant, and so forth are helpful) .

PROFESSIONAL HYGIENE

Because the esthetician's hands are in close contact with the client during the treatment, it is very important that she wash her hands with an antiseptic soap before ever touching the client's face and after each handling of an unsterilized object. All instruments and treatment accesssories must be disinfected with alcohol or an antiseptic immediately before use.

TIPS ON THE PSYCHOLOGY OF MAKING THE CLIENT COMFORTABLE

Once the work area is clean and properly arranged, the esthetician can admit her customer. While chatting with her to make her feel relaxed and comfortable, the esthetician can discreetly observe her makeup (the appearance of the skin under the foundation base, the harmony of the makeup, and so forth) . This preliminary observation can help guide the esthetician in choosing the correct products for treatment and eventually the appropriate makeup. Makeup does not hide a skin problem but can emphasize imperfections.

At the request of the esthetician, the client removes her dress, jewelry, and shoes, and puts on a smock. After hanging up her client's dress, the esthetician seats her in a chair. The back of the chair and footrest can be adjusted to a suitable height and angle for both the customer's comfort and the esthetician's convenience. The esthetician places a cover over her client so she does not become cold, lowers the straps of her brassiere to free her shoulders, and covers her head with a bonnet and headband so that her hair won't get wet.

After all these preparations are completed, it is time to fill out a questionnaire to open the customer's chart. It is necessary to be very diplomatic in order to obtain the maximum information possible, for the chart is very important in helping the esthetician know her customer better—her behavior, interests, and so forth. The chart also guides the esthetician in choosing the appropriate treatment and products, establishing a schedule of appointments, and determining the type of skin care the customer herself can adopt at home. The chart should be filled out, step by step, for the entire duration of the treatment and should be brought up to date regularly. For a suggested model of the customer's personal record, see the chart below.

CLIENT'S PERSONAL RECORD

Name: ____________ Address: ____________ Tel: ________

Date of Birth: ____________ Occupation: ____________ Tel: ________

Recommended by: ____________ Interests: ____________

Date	Skin Analysis	Products Suggested	Products Used
	Texture:	Milk:	
	Secretion:	Lotion Day cream:	
	Moisture:	Night cream:	
	Circulation:		Doctor:
		Liquids:	Surgical operations:
	Complexion:	Masks:	Drugs:
	Abnormalities:	Misc:	Allergies:

Date	Treatment	Date Next Appointment	Comments

8

Light Cleansing

The purpose of a light cleansing is to free the epidermis of makeup, dirt, and other substances (such as dead cells, secretions, and so forth) on the surface of the skin. It is important to clean the skin every morning and evening at home even if makeup is not used, for if the skin is not washed, it will lose its pretty complexion. Without this procedure, skin care products used at home may not be absorbed by the skin, and the esthetician may not get an accurate analysis of the skin in the studio.

Once the customer has been comfortably seated and the chart begun, the esthetician can start selecting the products to be used for the light cleansing—either an oil or special lotion for the eyes, a cleansing milk and lotion, and so forth.

LIPS

Give the customer a cleansing tissue to blot any excess lipstick. Then finish cleaning the lips with a cotton ball and cleansing milk.

EYES

Place a tissue under the eyelashes, and ask the customer to close her eyes. Dip a cotton swab in an oil or special cleansing lotion for the eyes, and use it to remove all makeup from the lashes. For very light makeup or for permanent lashes, the lotion is used. The oil is only used when heavy makeup has been applied. When the lashes are completely clean, moisten a cotton ball with oil or a special cleansing lotion for the eyes, and cleanse the eyelids, starting on the upper lid near the nose and working outward with a circular movement and coming back in toward the nose under the eye. The entire circular motion follows the palpebral and orbicular muscles of the eyelids. With a dry cotton ball repeat the same motion very, very gently to remove any surplus oil or lotion.

Removal of eye makeup

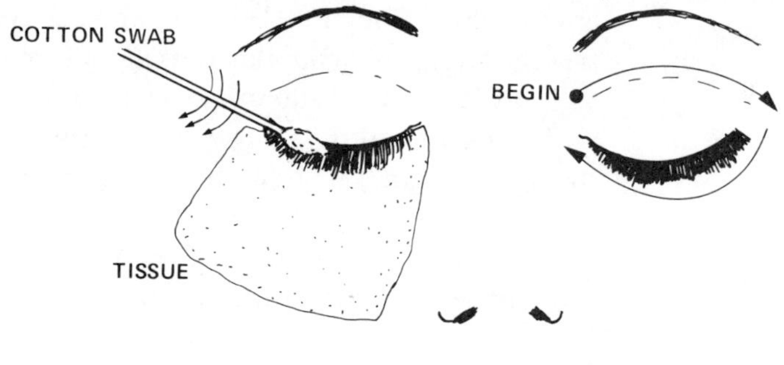

DÉCOLLETÉ, NECK, AND FACE

After selecting the appropriate cleansing milk, pour a small quantity of the milk into a cup and apply with the fingers to the face, neck, and décolleté using a circular motion to produce a good emulsion. Soak two muslin lamellae or special cleansing sponges in warm water and squeeze carefully. Place the cleansing pads between the fingers in such a way that the sponge is held by the index and little fingers and the part to be used by the esthetician rests in front of the middle and ring fingers.

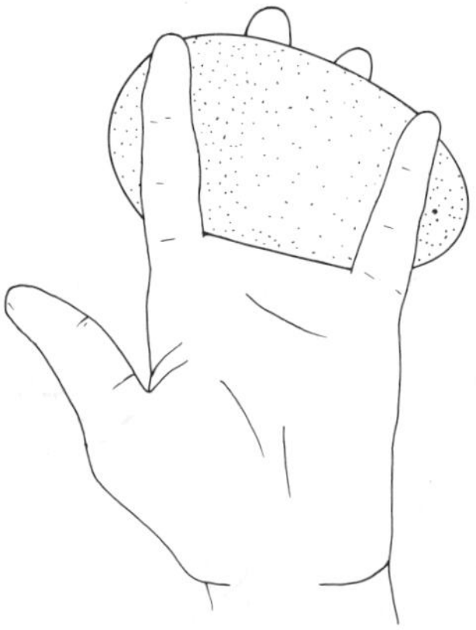

Using three circular effleurage movements, begin cleansing the décolleté at the base of the sternum (breastbone) in the hollow between the breasts, and work up from the shoulder towards the neck. Always using effleurage movements, cleanse the neck three times from the top to the base without lifting the hands from the client's skin. Continue by cleansing the regions of the mentalis, the triangularis, the orbicular muscle of the upper lip and nasalis area. Still using circular effleurage, cleanse along the pyramidal, frontal, and temporal muscles, the upper and lower orbicular muscle of the eyelid and finish with the masseters (three times). See the figure on the opposite page.

Rinse the lamellae and repeat the entire procedure at least three times, using clean, warm water.

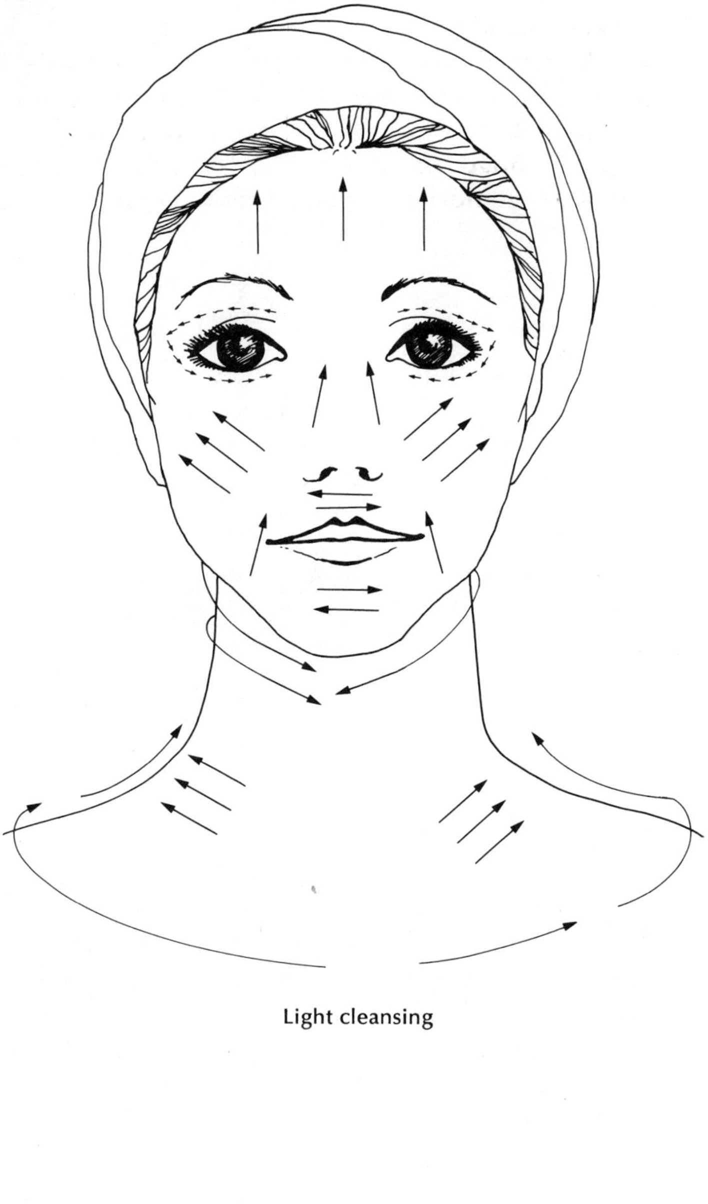

Light cleansing

ATOMIZATION

The entire cleansing operation is completed by a warm atomization using the appropriate apparatus. Fill the large cup with two thirds distilled water and one third floral lotion. The purpose of this very mild atomization of a warm, extremely fine water and lotion mist is to remove soluble or emulsified waste material that may still be present on the face, neck, or décolleté. A warm atomization also has an emollient and a relaxing effect.

The esthetician is now ready to analyze the skin and to continue filling out the client's chart.

9

Examination, Analysis, and Skin Care Recommendations

We have now arrived at the most important aspect of treatment: the analysis of the skin. The choice of treatment and products is based on the results of this examination. In Chapter 5, we described normal, dry, oily, and aging skins, but these are not the only characteristics the esthetician looks for in analyzing the skin. By themselves, these particular criteria are incomplete, since they are based only on the relative presence or absence of sebaceous secretions. Thus, it would not be correct to base an entire esthetic treatment on these criteria. An examination is therefore conducted with a magnifying glass in order to discern details or imperfections that are barely visible to the naked eye but could eventually develop more fully. It is important to feel the skin as well, since certain imperfections may be revealed to the touch, such as flaccidity, roughness, coarseness.

The esthetician plays an extremely important role in prevention, so she must carefully record all significant observations on the client's chart (texture, secretions, hydration and so forth). Only after this thorough examination can she begin treatment and subsequently prepare her recommendations.

Examination of the Skin

Important Observations	Distinctive Characteristics
TEXTURE:	
Delicate	Smooth, regular texture; invisible ostia; transparent (especially the eyelids), fragile appearance; sensitive; very soft to the touch
Normal	Fairly regular texture, neither too fine nor too coarse; visible ostia; supple, smooth to the touch
Coarse	Irregular, coarse texture; dilated ostia if caused by secretion and a tendency toward roughness; regular ostia if due to hereditary or racial traits; very solid appearance
Mixed	Middle of the face shiny with dilated ostia, usually rather coarse skin texture; rest of the face is normal, dry, or alipoidic
SECRETION:	
Hypolipoidic or alipoidic	Ostia more or less invisible; skin appearance rough, hard, worn, and parchmentlike with wrinkles and, frequently, fine scales
Normal	Ostia usually visible, but not dilated; middle portion of the face slightly more oily but not shiny; skin supple and contains no blackheads
Oily	Shiny as though wet; ostia large and frequently comedones are present; skin texture usually coarse

Important Observations	Distinctive Characteristics
Skin with a comedo condition	Same appearance as oily skin but with more comedones, blocked ostia, and oxidized sebum (blackheads) ; the more comedones the less oily the face looks because sebum is prevented from being secreted
Asphyxial	Irregular texture, coarse, unpleasant to the touch; sebum blocked and skin dry with milium nodules present
Acneic	Comedones; asphyxial conditions with inflammation and infection; scars. Acne is not contagious but easily spreads over the body of the person affected NEVER TOUCH—MEDICAL CONDITION
HYDRATION:	
Superficial dehydration	Scaling, dartre, pruritis (itching) ; small wrinkles around the eyes; slightly rough to the touch; lacking suppleness; exfoliation of the skin
Severe dehydration	Cracks in the skin, wrinkles; skin tends to be flaccid (flabby) , lacking in tone
CIRCULATION:	
Blotchy (telangiectasia; couperose)	Capillaries permanently dilated and visible, particularly around the cheeks, and nose, especially the nostrils
Diffuse redness (erythrosis)	Permanent or temporary diffuse redness; poor circulation; frequently blotchy
Rosacea (acne rosacea)	Acne with facial flushing, papules, and pustules NEVER TOUCH—MEDICAL CONDITION
COMPLEXION:	
Mixed	Asphyxial skin; coarse, oily, dull coloration
Faded	Alipoidic; appearance of general fatigue; autointoxication (e.g., cellular waste materials not eliminated or only poorly eliminated)
Bilious	Yellowish, oily skin

Examination of the Skin (*continued*)

Important Observations	Distinctive Characteristics
Pale	Waxy pallor (internal causes)
Dull	Dull coloration (internal causes)
ALLERGIES:	According to the client's descriptions and reactions
MISCELLANEOUS ANOMALIES:	
Circulation	Angiomas ("wine spots"); spider angiomas, also called nevus araneus (red circumscribed lesions with small capillaries radiating outward, resembling the legs of a spider); ruby spots (very small angiomas) NEVER TOUCH—MEDICAL CONDITION
Pigmentation	Hyperpigmentation: an increase in the quantity of pigment in the skin; freckles; chloasma: yellowish brown patches, which can occur in pregnancy; circles around the eyes Hypopigmentation: insufficient pigment (albinism) Dyschromia: any disorder in the pigmentation of the skin Vitiligo: discolored, white patches with regular contours. White spots due to the sun; liver spots; aging spots NEVER TOUCH—MEDICAL CONDITIONS
Hair	Pilosis: racial, hereditary Hypertrichosis: excessive growth of hair Hirsutism: abnormally long and abundant hair
Blemishes	Aqueous pockets (retaining water under the eyes), dilated ostia, milia, chapped areas, double chin. Can be treated by esthetics. Oily pockets (under the eyes), keratosis pilaris, cysts, xanthelasma (yellowish spots or patches due to lipoid deposits), scars (keloid or others), nevi (flat or raised), flat or common wart, verruca senilis (a flat, greasy wart usually seen in elderly people) NEVER TOUCH—MEDICAL CONDITIONS

It is important to study all these conditions in order to treat only those that apply to esthetics. Obviously, the examination of the skin is of the utmost importance; by assembling all of the different kinds of information on the client's record during the analysis of her skin, the esthetician will be in a position to provide a safe and useful treatment. If she feels it is necessary, the esthetician may even direct her client to a dermatologist.

By studying the flaws in the epidermis according to a predetermined method, the esthetician will be able to collect many observations, which may seem unrelated but which, in fact, depend on a common denominator. With the examination and case record completed, treatment may begin and a skin care plan prepared. The latter contains advice for the client about certain products, which may be used at home, and directions for their use. The esthetician must be honest and conscientious. She should recommend only those products that are absolutely necessary. Forced and exorbitant sales only serve to alienate customers from the institute. A sample skin care plan follows.

SKIN CARE RECOMMENDATIONS

Name: ______________________________

EVENINGS:

Remove eye makeup with ______________________________

Cleanse your face with ______________________________, rinse with warm water and then complete cleansing with your ______________________________ ______________ lotion.

Apply your ______________________________ treatment cream to your face and neck __________ times a week.

MORNINGS:

Cleanse just as in the evenings using your ______________________________ ______________ cleansing milk and follow with your ______________ ______________ lotion.

Apply a ______________________________ protection cream and then follow with your makeup, if desired.

REGULAR CARE:

________ times per week, following a thorough cleansing with ______________ ______________________________, apply the entire contents of a ________ ______________________________ ampul, followed by a ______________ ______________________________ mask.

SPECIAL TREATMENTS:

Eyes:

Neck:

Hand care:

Scalp:

Sun products:

Therapy: (acne, pimples, remoisturizing, color)

Your esthetician: ______________________________

Date	Treatment	Date Next Appointment	Comments

10

The Facial Massage: Methods and Effects

Massages can be performed for esthetic or therapeutic purposes. In this book, we will discuss esthetic massage, specifically of the face, neck, and décolleté.

To give a good massage that is not harmful, the esthetician must be sure that all of her movements follow the direction of the muscle fibers. This is the reason we studied the muscles and their functions earlier in this book. The muscles of the head and neck are composed of very fine fibers and are therefore very delicate. They can sag quite easily. A massage is able to stimulate blood circulation, which enhances blood flow to the skin and subcutaneous muscles. Improved circulation provides more oxygen and nutrients to the skin while removing more waste materials. Massaging also helps the skin absorb the active products contained within creams or serums.

The purpose of a massage is to restore the skin or to retain, for as long as possible, the skin's youthful condition and radiance. The various methods of massage for the face, neck, and décolleté will be explained in the following pages. Some of the products to use in performing facial massage are the oily serums, special massage creams, and biological creams.

AREA TO BE MASSAGED WITH THE APPROPRIATE TECHNIQUE

Décolleté (Effleurage)

Using three circular effleurage movements, begin massaging the décolleté at the base of the sternum (breastbone) in the hollow between the breasts, and work up from the shoulders toward the neck. Keep thumbs in front, hands in the back, pressing behind the ears, and slide down the sternum with the thumbs and index fingers applying a slight pressure (three times).

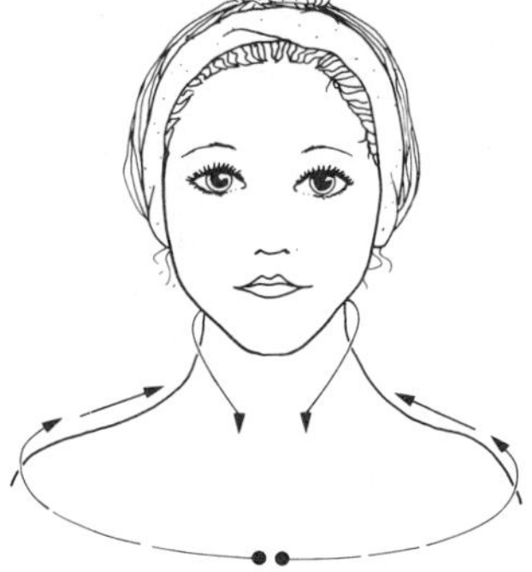

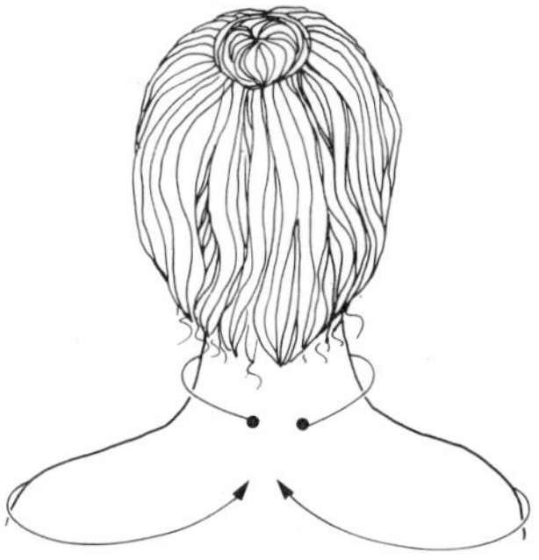

Trapezius

Apply light pressure sliding down; increase pressure moving back up.

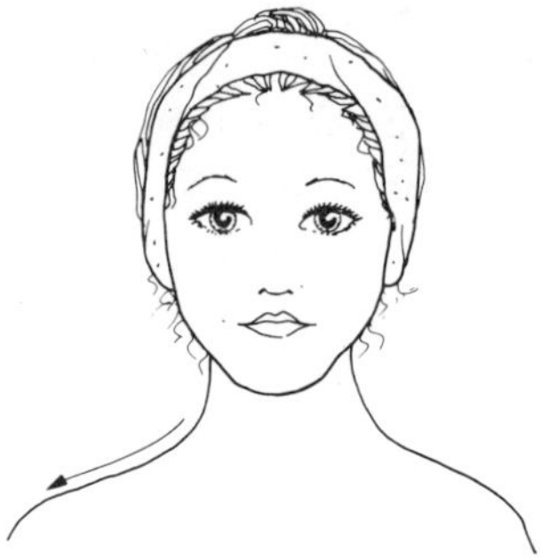

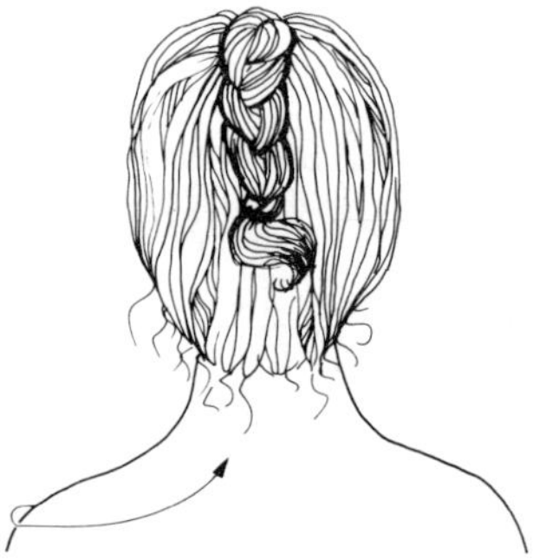

Nape of the Neck

With thumbs extended outward, massage in a semicircular motion.

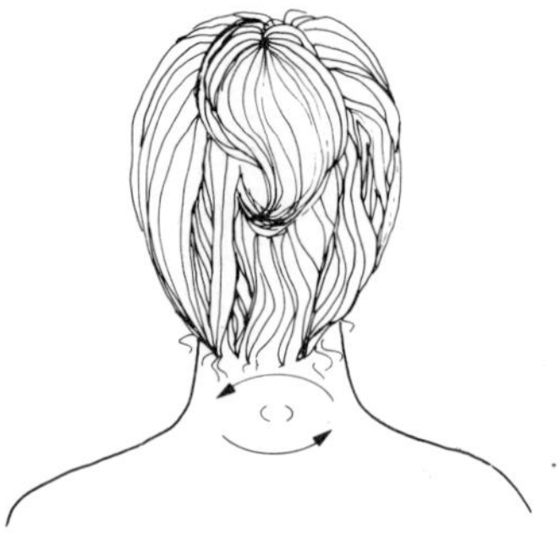

Neck

Massage with palm and fingers extended, work downward on the neck and then upward (three times) .

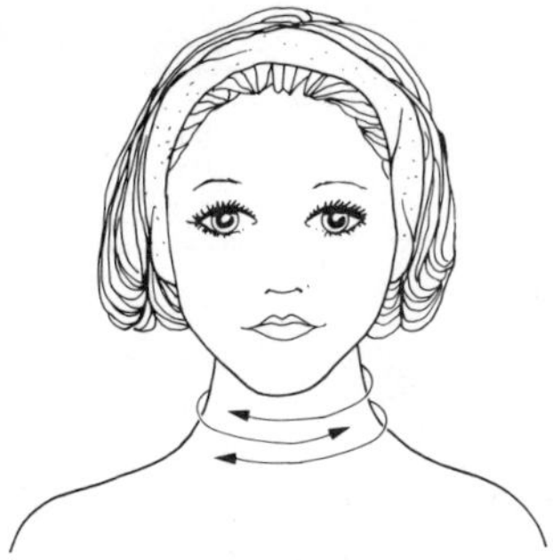

Sternum

With thumb and index finger, work downward, simultaneously, on both sides.

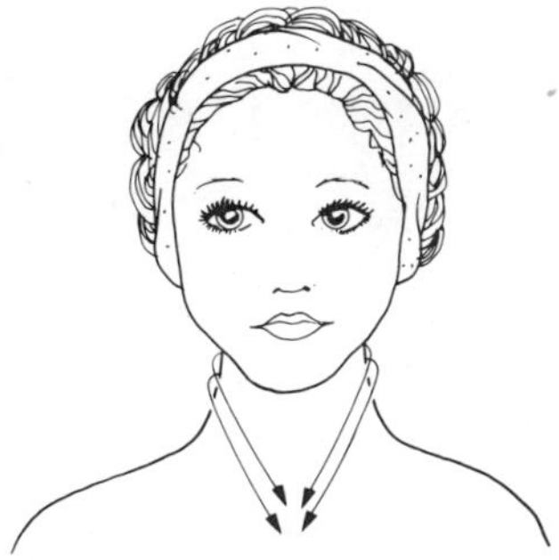

Masseters

Starting at the chin with hands in a conic position, move up to the eyes; then separate the hands, and move to the sides of the face.

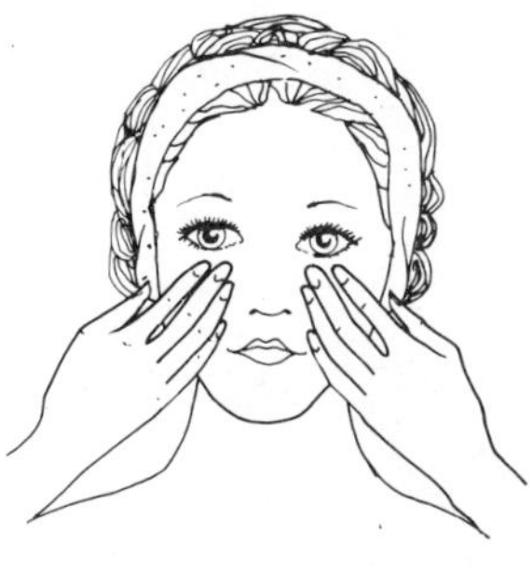

The arrows shown in the drawing below show the directions in which the hands should move.

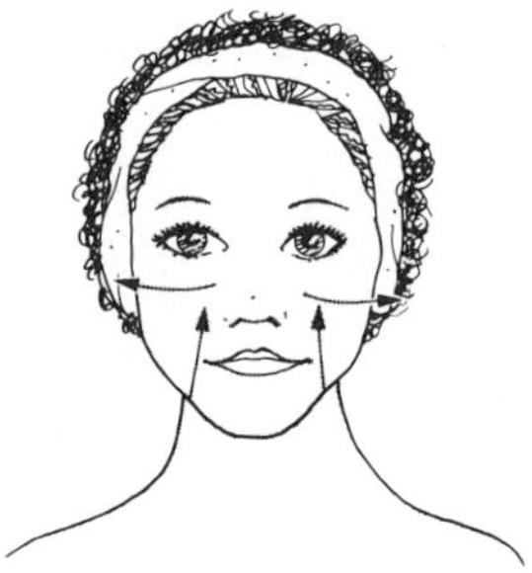

Triangularis of the Lips—Superficial and Deep Quadratus Muscles

With the index and middle fingers, move up the nasolabial furrow along both sides of the nose, and then press slightly with all the fingers on the forehead.

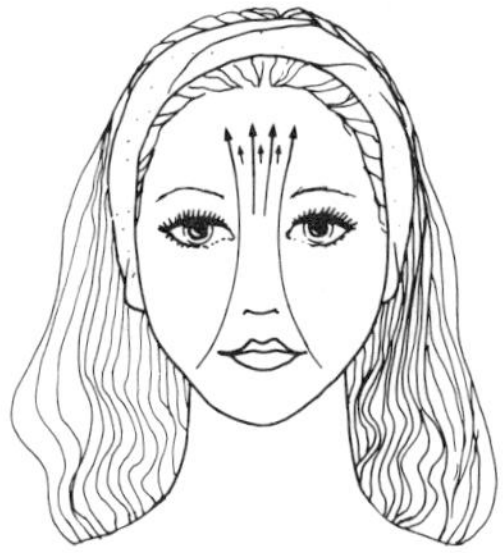

Orbicular Muscle of the Lips and the Zygomaticus Major

With the index and ring fingers, start at the center and move sideways to the corners of the mouth; then join all the fingers and effleurage up the zygomaticus.

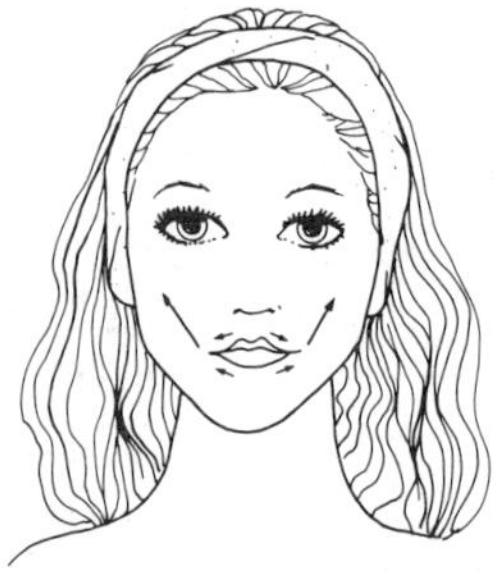

Transverse of the Nose

With the middle fingers of both hands bent, effleurage up and down each side of the nose.

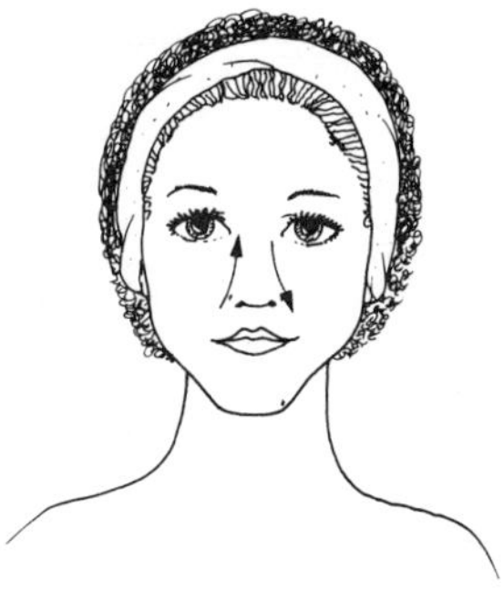

Orbicular Muscle of the Eyelid

Starting at the inside corners of the eyes, move with the index and ring fingers to the outside corners, and then join all the fingers and effleurage toward the temporalis.

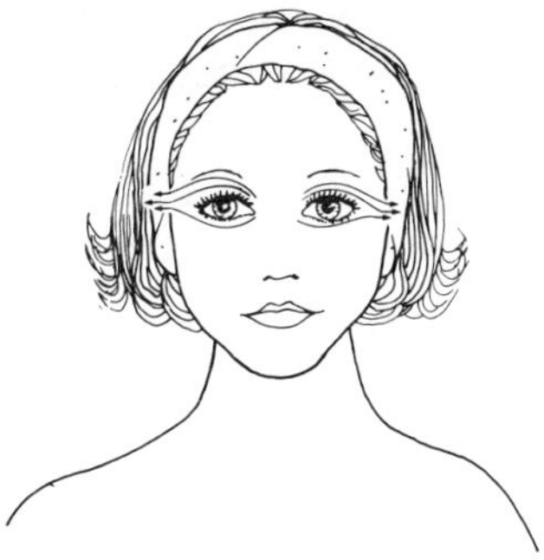

Pyramidalis, Frontal and Temporal

Alternating the hands, press slightly with the heel of one hand, and move with a continuous motion toward the fingertips; without losing contact, repeat the motion with the other hand.

In order to create an impression of continuity, the hands should follow each other without stopping.

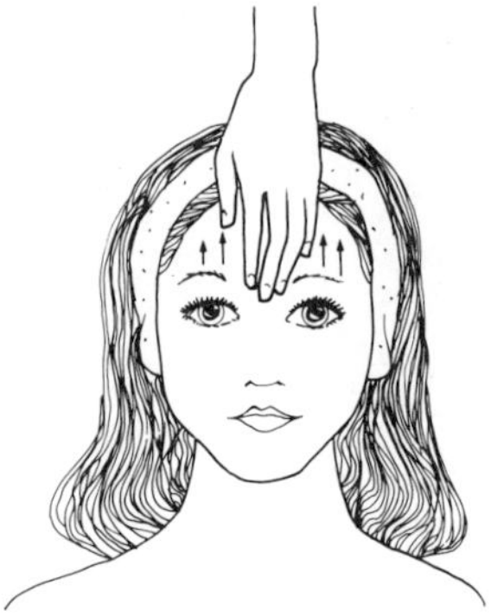

MOVEMENTS OF MASSAGE

Fingertip Pressures

Apply circular pressure on the masseters and zygomaticus with the middle finger.
Use a flicking upward motion on the masseters and zygomaticus with the middle fingers.
Apply circular pressure on the triangularis and the orbicular of the eyelids with the middle finger.
Use a flicking upward motion on the triangularis and the orbicular of the eyelids with the middle finger.

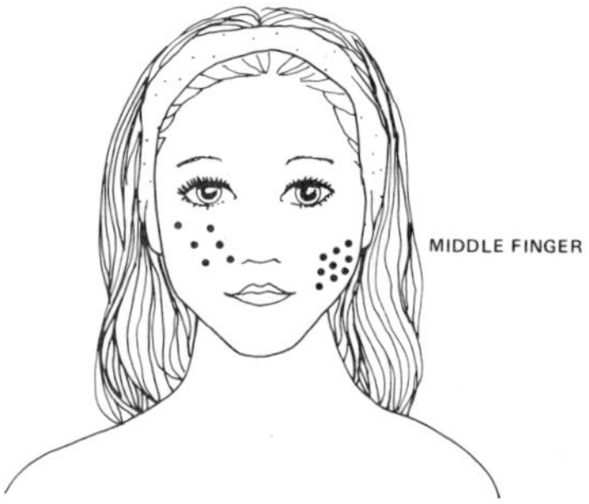

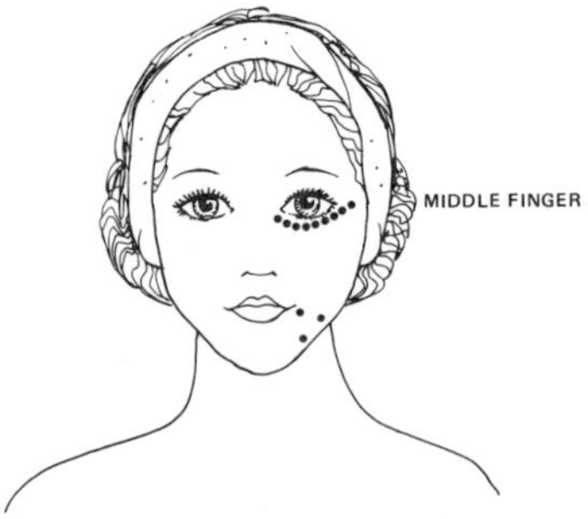

Pinching

Small Jacquets
Large Jacquets
Antiwrinkle pinching; with the thumb and middle finger, pinch while sliding over each wrinkle.

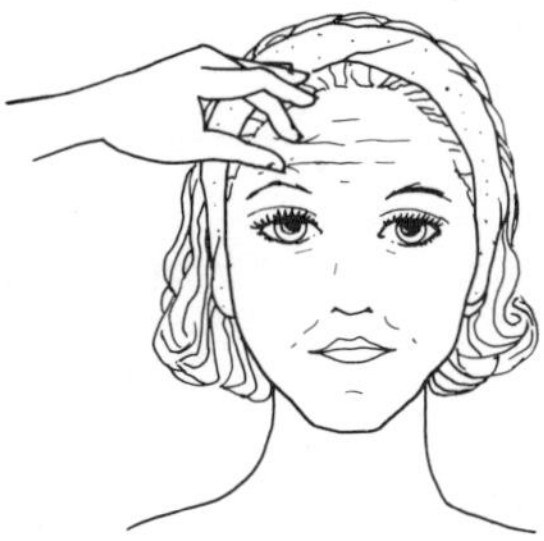

Cupping

Cupping is done by pressing the palms of the hands firmly on the forehead and chin.

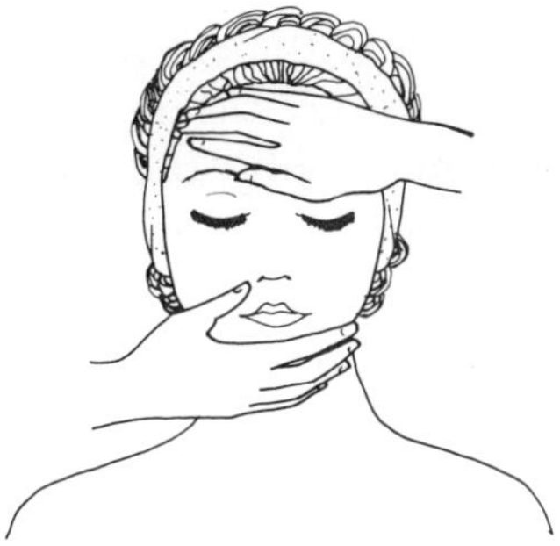

On the cheeks, press firmly with both hands to create a suction.

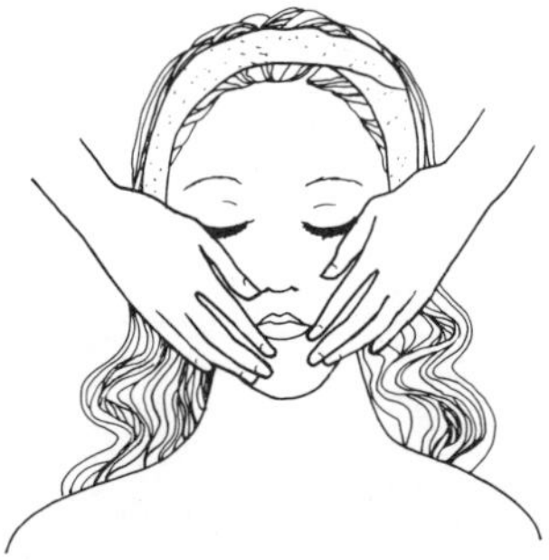

Foulage

Hold the layers of the skin firmly with the middle and index fingers of one hand; smooth and slide the index finger of the other hand over the wrinkles.

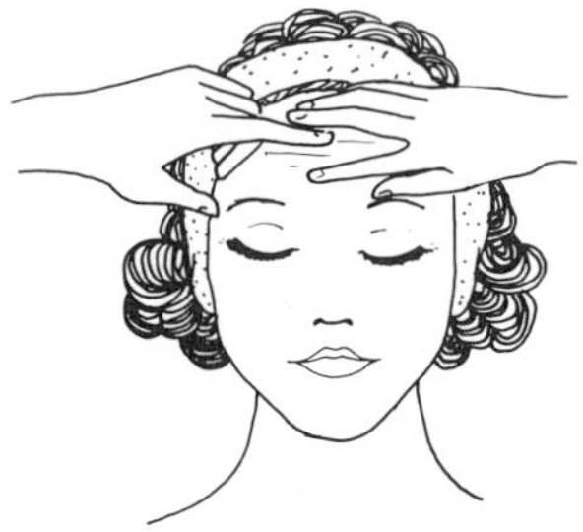

Eye Treatment

Effleurage around the eyes.
Treatment for crow's-feet consists of effleurages applied in a figure-eight pattern. Hold the layers of the skin around the outer portion of the eye firmly with the middle and index fingers of one hand. Move the middle finger of the other hand in a swirling motion around the crow's-feet, pressing lightly. Pause and repeat the procedure. The purpose of this movement is to smooth out the lines of the crow's-feet. Particular care must be taken to prevent any products from going into the eyes and always to move with very light and delicate movements around the eyes.

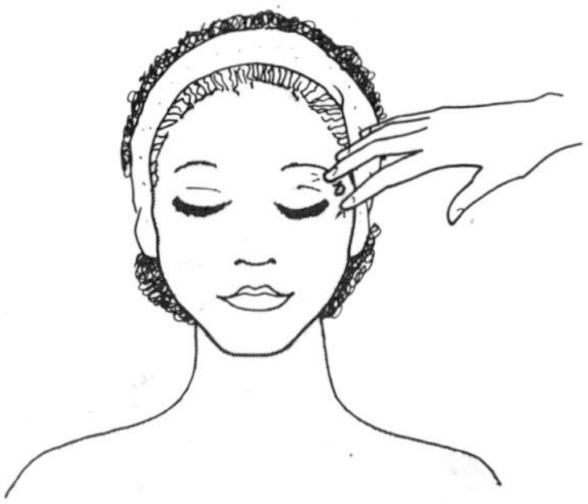

Final Effleurage Combination

Do a combination effleurage, moving up over the masseters, orbicular of the eyelids, and pyramidalis nasi, joining the hands over the forehead; then slide outward over the temporals and down the cheeks, fan out fingers, and move back upward and outward over the masseters.

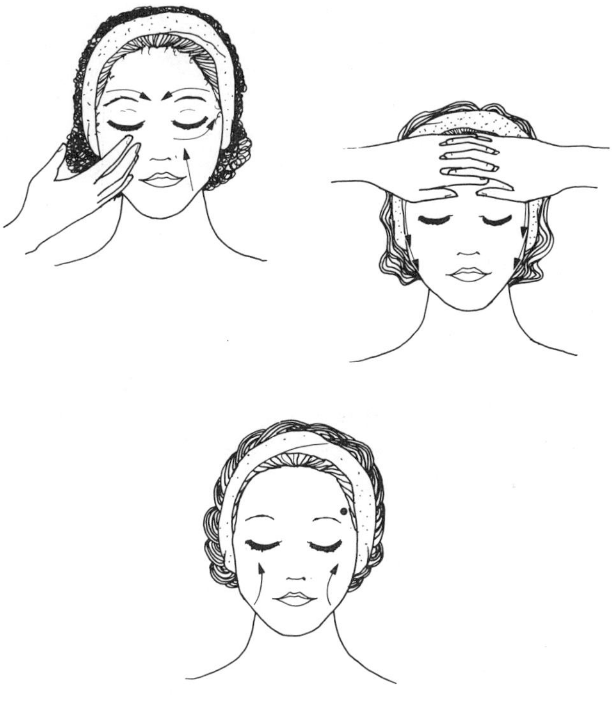

THE EFFECTS OF MASSAGE

Effleurages

All massages must begin and conclude with effleurage, which are movements consisting of moving the palm of the hand or the fingers over the surface of the skin but exerting very little pressure, so that the skin does not move. Effleurage movements have a soothing and relaxing effect and assist blood and lymphatic flow.

Effleurage permits the esthetician to be in contact with her client and thus to relax her, win her confidence, and mentally condition her for receiving other massage manipulations. It also gives the esthetician an opportunity to evaluate the condition of the tissues.

Fingertip Pressures

Circular pressures are small, very precise but firm circles, usually performed with the middle finger. For the nose, the thumb is used. The fingers never slide; rather, the skin, because of its mobility, slides over the deeper layers.

Fingertip flicking pressure is performed with the middle finger. The rhythm can vary (regular or irregular staccata) . Circular and flicking pressures have a toning, stimulant effect, rendering the skin more supple.

Pinching

Small Jacquet pinches are performed with the thumb and second joint of the index finger in all directions. They are particularly suitable for dry skin. They activate circulation (far better distribution of blood at the periphery) and make the skin more supple. Large Jacquet pinches are performed on oily skin only without cream or other products. They serve to free the follicles of excess sebum. (The Jacquet pinch takes its name from Dr. Jacquet, a well-known dermatologist.)

The antiwrinkle pinch is done with the thumb and middle finger on all wrinkles in order to increase local blood supplies and to make the wrinkles swell, preparing the skin to absorb the treatment product.

Slapping, Petrissages, and Percussion

Slapping is done with the middle fingers on the masseters, triangularis, and the quadratus muscles. It is also done with the hands for a double chin, for it exerts a firming effect and helps in-increase the local blood supply.

Petrissages, or percussion, are short, rhythmical tapping movements, which vary with the position of the hand. The so-called pianotements are produced with the palmar surface of the fingers. When applied by rolling with all the fingers under the chin, the pianotements exert an effect on the facial oval by increasing the muscle tone and contractility.

Cupping

The purpose of cupping is to increase the local blood supply, especially in blemished skin. Press the palm of the hand firmly on the forehead and chin and then on the cheeks.

Foulage

Foulage is performed by holding the layers of the skin firmly with the middle and index fingers of the left hand while smoothing and sliding the middle finger of the right hand, with a slight pressure, over the wrinkles. Do not exert any pressure on the hyoid bone of the neck.

Conclusion

A massage should be concluded by combining the effleurage manipulations used at the start. This has a very soothing effect. The esthetician must remember that a facial massage must always be performed very calmly, without unnecessary noise and in a pleasant and comfortable atmosphere. The esthetician stands behind her client's chair with her feet slightly apart. She must never move during a massage. Her movements and gestures should always be graceful and elegant.

The esthetician's hands should be cleaned with a bactericidal soap before and after each massage. During the massage her hands should be warm and dry. She should remove the massage cream from the jar with a spatula and never put her fingers directly into the jar. If she uses a serum, the esthetician should empty it into a small sterilized crucible or into the hollow of her hand, which has been washed with alcohol. The esthetician should always have her entire hands in contact with the surface to be massaged. She should never interrupt a massage or show any hesitation. The manipulations must always be well integrated and connected. Pressure should never be applied to the hyoid bone.

Always perform very light, delicate massages or effleurage on delicate, strained, fine, sensitive, or blotchy skin. Never massage acneic skin. All massage movements on the face must be performed with a light, soft, but sure touch. The specific manipulations must be selected according to the type, appearance, and quality of the client's skin with consideration as well for her age and psychological state.

11

Electrical Equipment

THE USE OF ELECTRICITY IN ESTHETICS

Electricity is one form of energy found in the universe. For many of us, electricity will always remain a mystery, probably because it is invisible, and its presence can only be verified by the effects it produces. It is important to define its components at this time.

First, though, we will discuss the concept of matter, and then we will be able to understand the chemical and electrical phenomena that affect matter.

Matter

The term *matter* is a synonym for all existing substances (solid, liquid, gaseous). Matter can be subdivided into two categories: simple and complex.

Simple matter: composed of just one substance, for example, iron, sulfur, oxygen.

Complex matter: composed of two or more different substances. The bonds uniting these substances can be broken by a chemical reaction, isolating each individual component. For example, table salt is composed of chloride and sodium, and water of hydrogen and oxygen.

Matter is made up of particles so tiny that they are not visible with even the strongest microscope. These infinitely small particles are called atoms.

Structure of the Atom

Long ago, the atom was thought to be the smallest particle of matter. This idea was conveyed through the word *atom* itself, which comes from the Greek *atomos* (indivisible). Now it has been established that there are even smaller particles, which are the atomic components.

An atom is composed of a central core called a *nucleus,* which is positively charged, and an outer portion containing electrons, which are negatively charged.

The Nucleus. The nucleus is composed of two types of particles: protons and neutrons. Protons and neutrons are about the same size and have a similar mass. Protons carry a positive electric charge; neutrons carry no charge, or are neutral. Nevertheless, the neutrons prevent the protons from repelling each other and keep the nucleus intact.

The Electron. The electron is an extremely light, negatively charged particle which rotates around the nucleus. Electrons occupy various concentric orbits around the nucleus.

The attraction between the positive protons of the nucleus and the negative electrons distinguishes the atom as a complete entity. One of the laws of physics states that a positive will attract a negative and that a positive and negative will nullify each other. Conversely, a positive (or negative) will repel another positive (or negative). Thus, opposite charges attract and like charges repel each other.

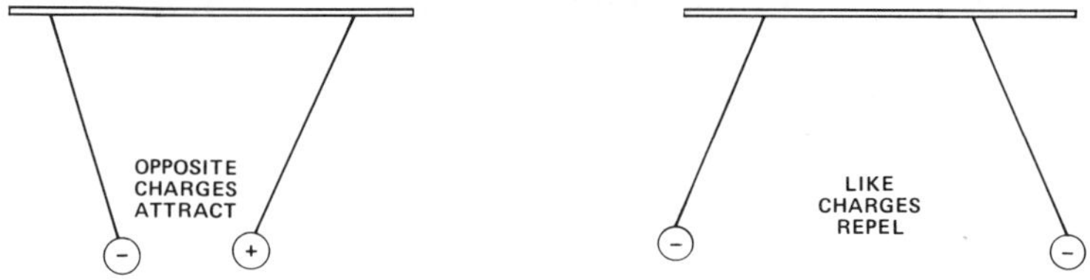

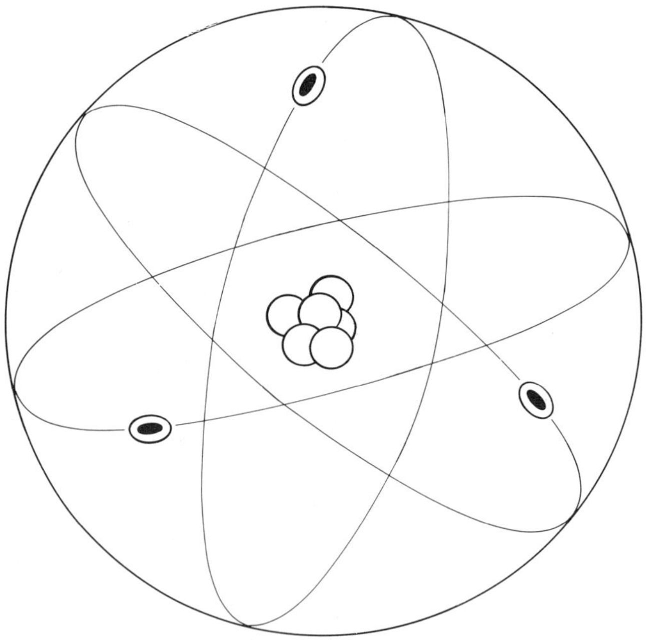

The atom

Neutral Atoms and Ions

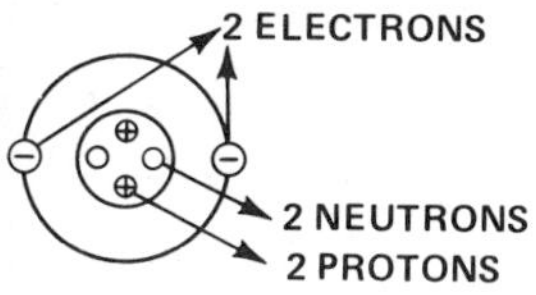

An atom of a particular element always contains a fixed number of protons. If it contains an equal number of protons and electrons, the atom has no overall charge because the positive charges cancel the negative charges. Such an atom is neutral. Helium is an example of a neutral atom.

Under certain chemical or physical conditions, a neutral atom can gain or lose electrons. If it loses one or more electrons, the number of protons (which is always fixed for a given element) becomes greater than the number of electrons, and thus there are more positive charges, giving the atom an overall positive charge. A positively charged atom is called a positive ion, or cation. Likewise, if an atom gains one or more electrons, the overall charge becomes negative, and the atom is then called a negative ion, or anion.

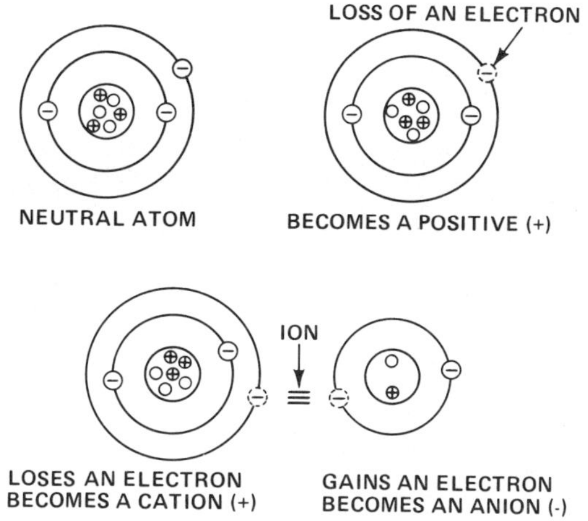

Molecule

Neutral atoms do not usually exist in a free state, as such, nor are positive or negative ions normally found in the universe. In reality we usually find neutral molecules, which are formed by uniting:

1. Either two or more neutral atoms
   (For example, oxygen exists as an oxygen molecule, which is composed of two oxygen atoms.)

2. Or a positive ion with a negative ion.
(For example, table salt is actually made of a molecule of sodium chloride (NaCl), which is the union of a sodium ion (Na^{+}) with a chloride ion (Cl^{-}).

The preferred state of matter in the universe is generally that which is the most stable. Some neutral atoms are actually more stable if they gain or lose one or more electrons. When these atoms enter each other's presence, they accommodate each other: one by giving up an electron (s) and the other by accepting it (them). Such is the case with sodium (Na), which is more stable if it loses an electron, and of chlorine (Cl), which is more stable with an extra electron.

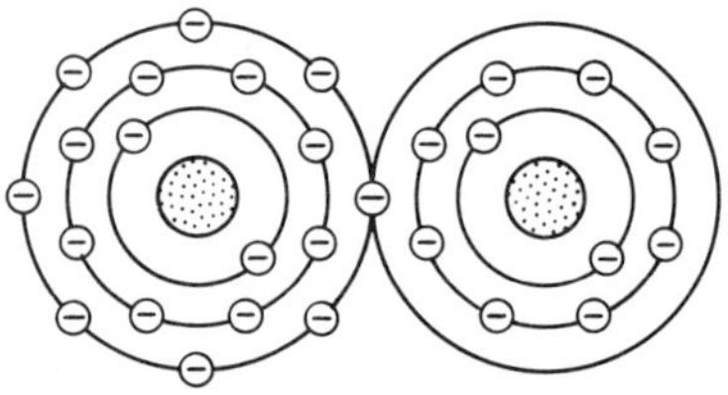

SALT MOLECULE
(NaCl)

It is the movement of electrons from one atom to another that constitutes an electrical current. In esthetics, several types of current are used for various forms of treatment. However, in this chapter we will discuss only the use of high-frequency current and galvanic current. We will study the aims and principles behind the use of these currents while explaining how the various instruments operate.

ELECTRICAL EQUIPMENT

Warm Atomizer

The electric atomizer was invented by Dr. Lucas Championnière (1843–1913). There have been many different types of warm atomizers, but all provide the same effect for the same purpose.

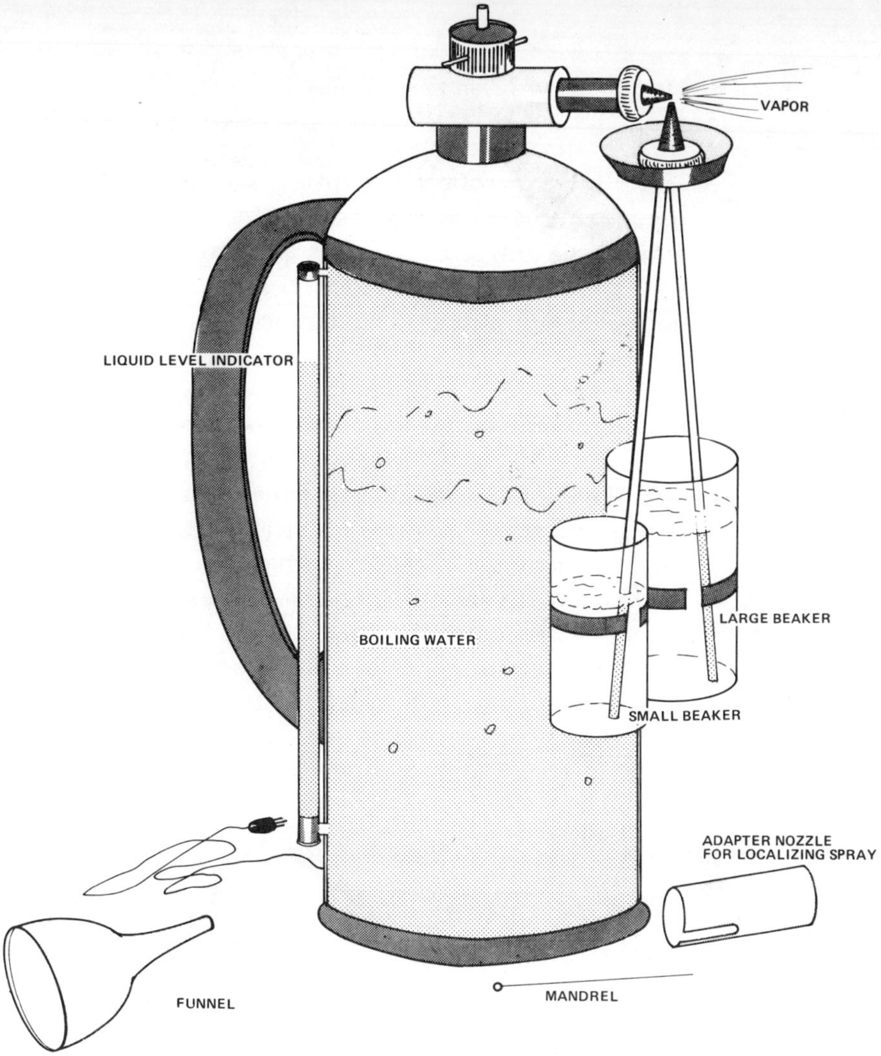

Purpose. Very gentle atomization of water or a lotion into a very warm, fine mist has a calming and emollient effect. It carries away soluble or emulsified waste products, which may be left on the face after cleansing.

Use. For all types of skin, always at the beginning of a treatment.

Instructions for Use. Unscrew the cap on the top of the instrument. Fill the reservoir up to the three-quarter mark with distilled or demineralized water, using a small funnel. Reclose the cap firmly. Fill the large beaker three quarters full with the distilled water or lotion that is to be atomized. (The small beaker serves only to collect the droplets from condensation.) Connect the apparatus to an electrical outlet. When the atomizer is warm and begins to work, release its spray for a few moments away from your client's face. If the atomizer sputters or spits, it is because it is not being held straight or it is defective.

Caution. Never let the boiler or metal portions of the atomizer come into contact with you or your client.

Note. Make certain that the openings from which the vapor and liquid escape are always clean so that the atomized material can pass through freely. The small openings of the apparatus can be opened up with a mandrel (a fine metal rod). There is a special adapter nozzle which can be used to limit or localize the area to be atomized. When the atomization is completed, take a tissue in which a hole has been made for the nose, and place it over the client's face. Pat dry starting at the eyes and then going to the forehead, chin, and cheeks. Never rub.

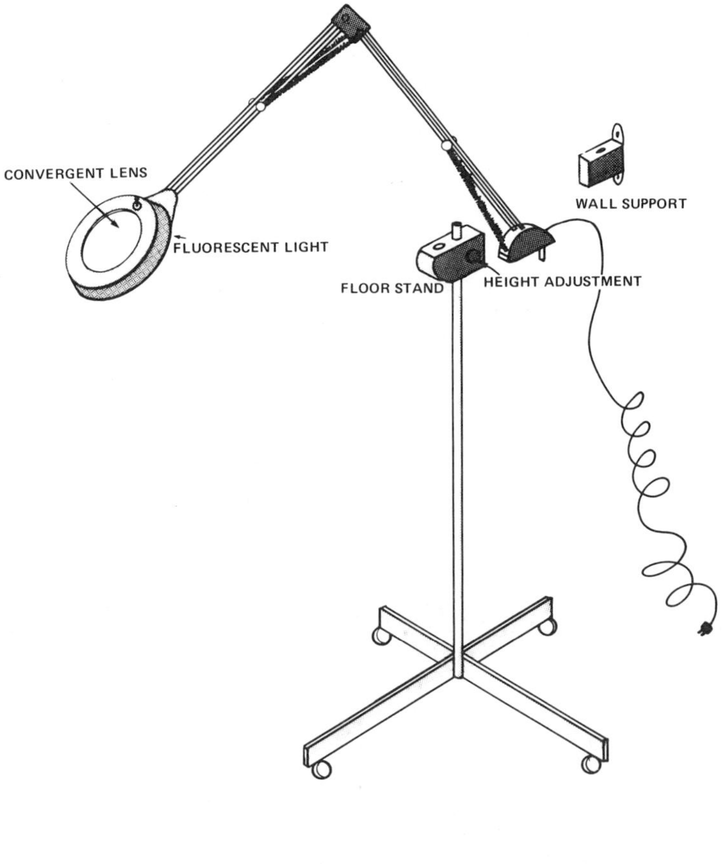

Magnifying Lamp

The magnifying lamp has a convergent lens that magnifies objects. The frame around the magnifying lamp is fitted with a fluorescent light that illuminates the surface being treated or examined.

The magnifying lamp is used in esthetics for examining the skin, extracting comedones, plucking eyebrows, and so forth. Depending on which attachment is used, the magnifying lamp can be located on a table, on the wall, or on a floor stand or be attached to different instruments. Its length and height are adjustable. (See illustration on opposite page.)

Warm Vaporizer

A warm vaporizer converts ordinary water vapor to a very fine mist, whereupon the water molecules divide (become ionized). This produces ozone, which also serves a purpose described below.

Properties of Ozone (O_3). Ozone (O_3) can be thought of as condensed oxygen. Ozone exists naturally in the atmosphere but in very small quantities. The ozone molecule is composed of three oxygen atoms, whereas molecules of normal oxygen contain only two oxygen atoms. In the air, ozone is produced by an electrical charge (lightning). The thickness of the ozone layer is also proportional to the ultraviolet radiation emitted by the sun; thus it acts as a protective covering for us. When ozone decomposes, it emits a mild ultraviolet ray that possesses remarkable physiological properties. The mist of an ozone vaporizer increases the circulation in the skin, which serves to enhance its nutrition and to eliminate wastes.

Purposes. The warm vaporizer may be used for several purposes:

Dilation of the ostia
Emollient
Preparation of the epidermis for removal of comedones
Mildly moisturizing
Increase of circulation in the skin

Activation of controlled peeling

Mild bactericidal effect

Scalp treatment

Use. For oily, acneic, coarse, or dehydrated skin, apply for 15 to 20 minutes at a distance of 8 inches. For normal skin, apply for 15 to 20 minutes at a distance of 10 inches. For delicate, sensitive, or blotchy skin, apply for 10 to 15 minutes at a distance of 12 to 15 inches.

Instructions for Use. Fill the bottle or reservoir up to the indicated level with distilled or demineralized water. Replace the cover carefully so that the water does not overflow when it begins to boil. Connect the apparatus to an electrical outlet.

Place the steam switch in the ON position. When the vapor starts to rise, place the ozone switch in the ON position (to produce ozonized vapor) . Direct the vapor toward the client's face from the correct distance and for the specified amount of time.

The warm vaporizer can also be used without ionized vapor, if desired. To do this, the ozone switch must be left in the OFF position, and then the vapor may be directed toward the client's face. This method is particularly recommended for the treatment of pigment spots.

Maintenance. The bottle or reservoir must be drained regularly one or two times a week. To eliminate calcium deposits, the bottle or reservoir should be cleaned frequently with vinegar and water. The latter mixture should be brought to a boil for 5 minutes and then allowed to stand for another 15 minutes to take effect. While this is being done, the spontex must be removed from the swivel head so that it does not acquire the odor of vinegar. Then rinse the water container with clear water.

Note. Some massage techniques can be performed under the warm vaporizer using a vitaminized cream. This facilitates the removal of comedones by softening them. It is very important to follow such a massage with a light cleansing (milk and lotion) because the cream present on the skin will interfere with the removal of the comedones and the remainder of the treatment if a therapeutic serum is to be used.

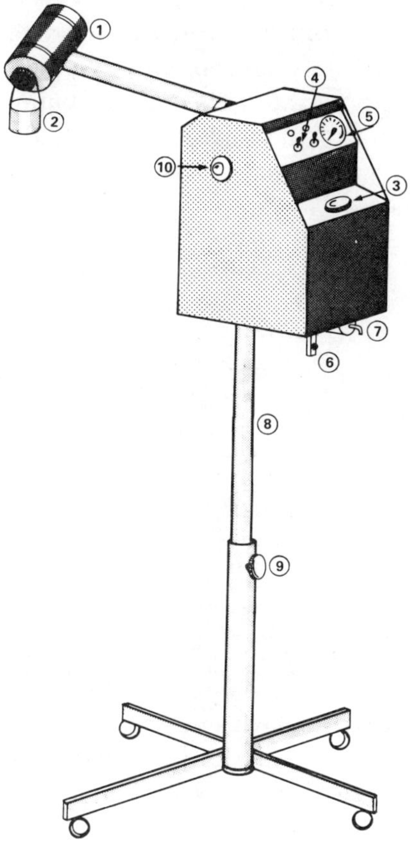

Warm vaporizer

1. swivel head
2. droplets collector
3. fill cap
4. vapor and ozone switch
5. automatic timer
6. reset button
7. drain
8. adjustable height stand
9. adjustment stop screw
10. pilot lamp

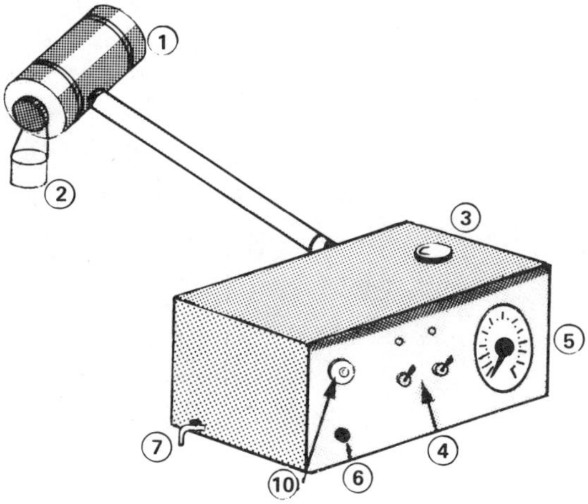

Portable warm vaporizer

High-Frequency Apparatus

High-frequency currents, used as early as 1897 by Professor d'Arsonval, are alternating currents. In other words, they change direction extremely rapidly, approximately several times per second. They can pass through the body without the person being aware of it. The repeated changes in the direction of high-frequency current have the effect of an internal massage acting on the nerves, the cells, and the muscles.

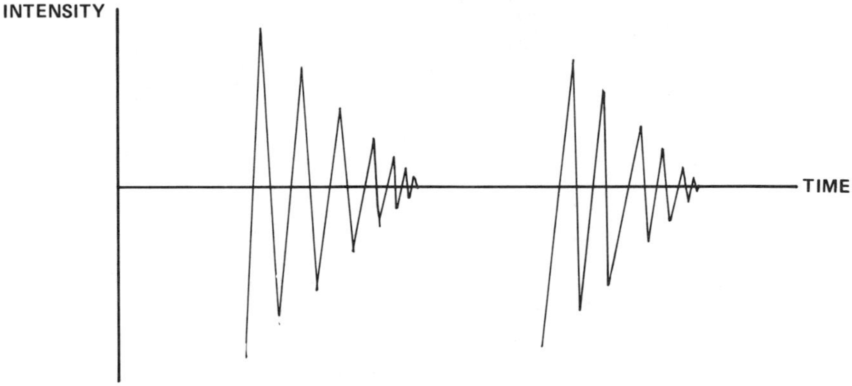

Properties. High-frequency currents have a very great penetrating power. They do not stimulate the muscles but produce a warming effect within the tissues. These currents possess an action that is specific to the electrode used to produce them. There are three types of rays produced by high-frequency currents, which again depend on the electrode used. The three types of rays are: violet, neon, and ultraviolet.

Violet Ray: A violet ray electrode is used for facial massage. Due to its revulsive effect, this electrode activates the circulation and improves tissue nutrition. It is also used after the removal of comedones because it releases ozone and thus has a mild bactericidal effect.

Neon (Pink) Ray: These electrodes exert the same effects as the violet ray electrodes except that they have a more gentle effect and therefore should be used for sensitive skins. They also exert a decongestant effect. They are particularly recommended for couperosed conditions and following electrolysis procedures.

Ultraviolet Ray: When a violet ray is passed through mercury vapor, it is transformed into an ultraviolet ray and is emitted through a quartz electrode. This electrode is used primarily for the bactericidal action of the ultraviolet ray. The ultraviolet ray is also used for tanning.

High-frequency currents can come into direct contact with the entire body by using a general discharge produced by a saturating electrode. The client holds the electrode in her hand for about five minutes. The entire body then becomes alternately charged and discharged.

Saturation: One of the best toning treatments. It regulates blood pressure, balances the organic functions and facilitates blood circulation.

Effleurage: A gentle treatment that enhances blood circulation. It is performed with a rotating motion always in the direction of the muscles, with the electrode always in contact with the client's skin.

Etincelage or Fulguration: After the removal of comedones, this technique helps serums penetrate into the skin, destroy bacteria, and tone the skin. The electrode is held above the skin and emits small sparks, which can be directed toward the area to be treated.

Indirect Massage: Activates the general circulation. Prepares the skin for active products and helps aqueous serums penetrate the skin. The client holds the spiral electrode in her hand, and the esthetician's hands become the active electrodes. Small pinching movements are made in all directions.

Directions for Use: After the apparatus has been plugged in, push the appropriate electrode down into the holder until it is firmly inserted inside the handle. Turn the switch of the apparatus to the ON position. Place the electrode on the client's face while taking care to keep a finger on the electrode so as to prevent a shock as it comes into contact with her face. Take the finger off and progressively increase the intensity according to the client's sensitivity. At the end of the treatment, gradually reduce the intensity and place the finger back on the electrode before lifting it off the client's face.

After each use, carefully clean the electrodes with a damp cloth. Before using any electrode, make sure it has been completely disinfected. If alcohol has been used as the disinfectant, make certain that there are no traces of it left on the electrode before turning on the apparatus.

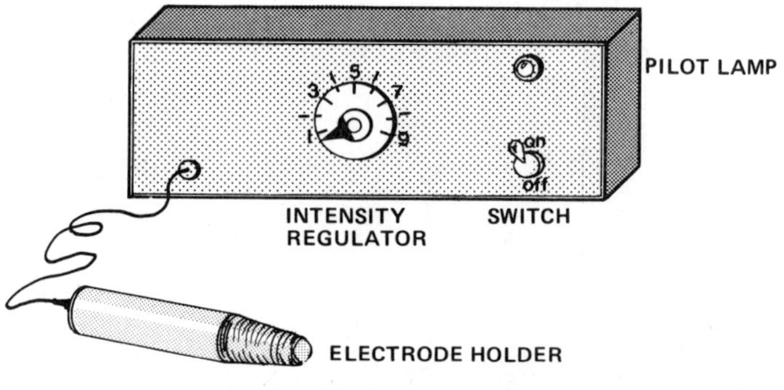

Different Types of Electrodes Used in Esthetics

Precaution. Metal point electrodes are never to be used in esthetics. They are reserved for medical use only.

Note. High-frequency currents with a higher intensity are also used for definitive depilation.

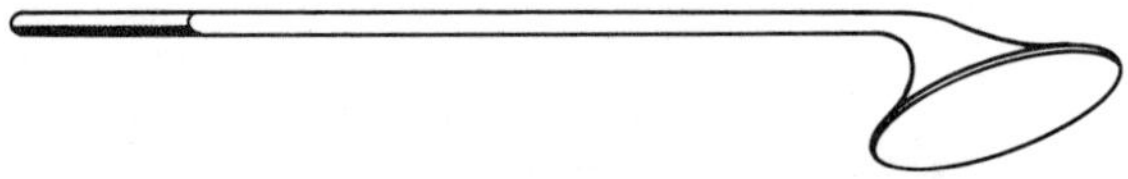

Violet electrode, wide surface, which is used for facial massage, effleurage, and etincelage

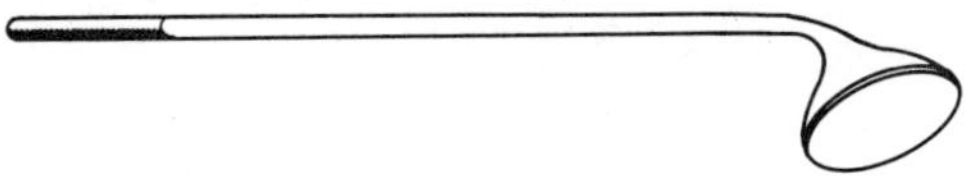

Neon electrode (pink ray electrode), small surface, which is used for facial massage, effleurage, and etincelage

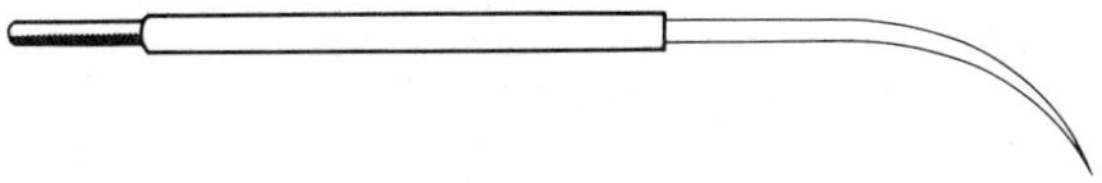

Glass point electrode, which is used for etincelage or fulguration

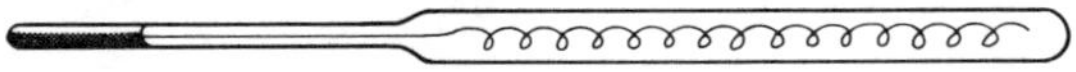

Spiral electrode, which is used for indirect massage and saturation

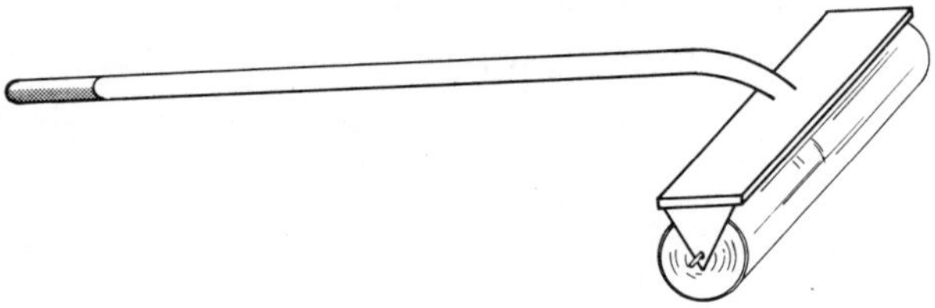

Neon or violet roller electrode, which is used for very mild massage

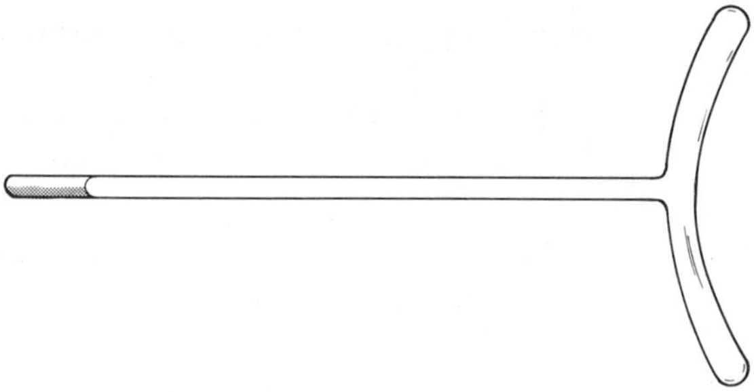

Neck electrode, which is used for effleurage

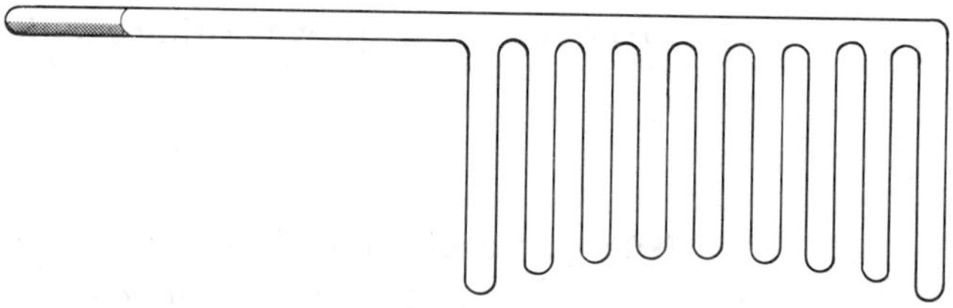

Comb electrode, which is used for scalp treatments. Never use with lotions containing alcohol.

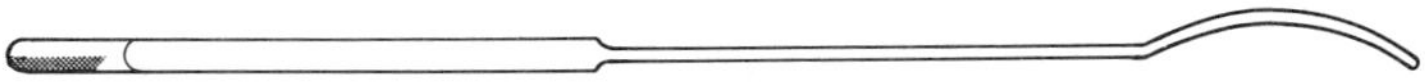

Eyelid electrode, which is often used over a tissue. This electrode has a very weak intensity.

Vacuum and Spray Apparatus

Spray Use.

Cold atomization, toning; always at the end of a treatment.

Galvanic douche (see Ionizing Galvanic Douche).

A combination of two instruments for the treatment of acne and dehydration; for cleansing and disincrustation in areas that are difficult to reach, such as the edges of the nose.

Diffused Spray: Used to vaporize aqueous serums or lotions and to soften facial masks at

	the end of a treatment in order to facilitate their removal. Also used to help water or lotion to be absorbed by the horny layer (imbibition).
Stream Sprayer:	Used for the galvanic douche, a combination of two instruments (see Ionizing Galvanic Douche).

Directions for Spray Use. Plug the apparatus into an electrical outlet. Fill one of the containers with water or the lotion to be atomized. Turn the switch of the apparatus to the ON position and direct the spray towards the client's face. The force of the spray may be regulated by turning the tip of the nozzle. The maximum force is obtained by covering the opening in the atomizer cap with your thumb.

Note. Never spray directly toward the nostrils as this may impair breathing. It is recommended that a shallow face pan be used for the galvanic douche.

Maintenance. To prevent the openings of the sprayer from becoming clogged, atomize clear water after each atomization of a serum or lotion.

Suction Use. To activate blood and lymphatic circulation in the tissues; to remove the skin's waste materials from the epidermis; to remove excess sebum from the pilosebaceous follicles; to facilitate the removal of comedones and to reduce wrinkles temporarily.

Directions for Suction Use. After the skin has been well prepared by a light and deep cleansing (gentle peeling), the esthetician places the client under the warm vaporizer before proceeding, with the help of the aspirator, to

1. Remove excess sebum from the pilosebaceous follicles
2. Remove cutaneous waste materials from the epidermis

3. Massage by aspiration to activate the circulation
4. Remove comedones
5. Fill out the wrinkles

These procedures prepare the skin to better absorb a serum or other active products. Massage movements must always be performed in the same direction as the muscle fibers.

Place a cupping glass on the muscle, cover the opening with a finger until the area just begins to redden, then take the finger away before moving the cupping glass so that the capillaries will not be damaged. Particular care must be taken to massage gently under the eyes and around the mouth.

The small flat cupping glass is intended for the treatment of wrinkles. For that purpose, the esthetician must always work in the pattern of an "X" and never pull at the skin. Using the small comedone-extracting cupping glass, comedones are removed or their removal is facilitated. Comedones should never be forced out by a cupping glass as forcing will leave marks on the face.

Note. The larger the cupping glass, the weaker the suction. The smaller the mouth of the cupping glass, the stronger the force. It is important to avoid overly long or intense suction. Suction must not be applied to couperosed skin.

Maintenance. Wash the cupping glasses with soap and water and always disinfect with alcohol or a bactericidal agent before using.

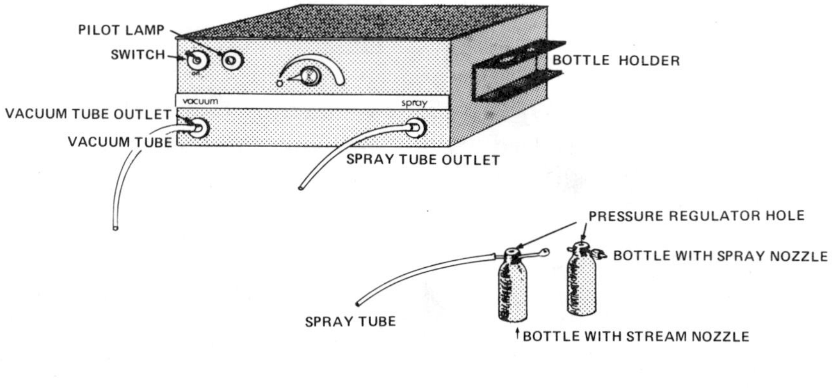

Different Cupping Glasses Used with the Vacuum Apparatus

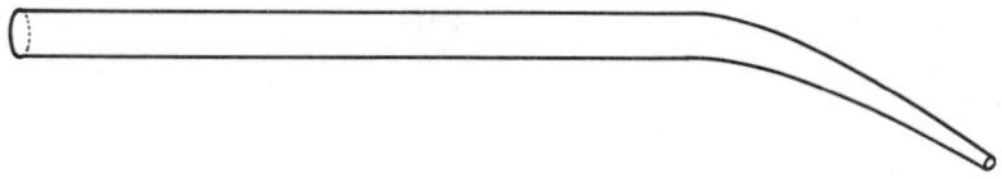

Comedo extractor cupping glass

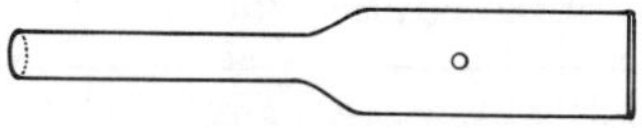

Antiwrinkle cupping glass

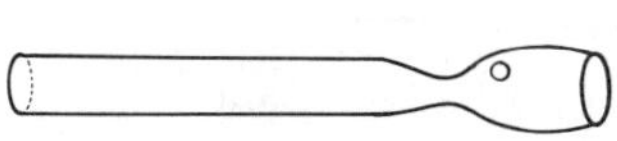

Sebum extractor cupping glass

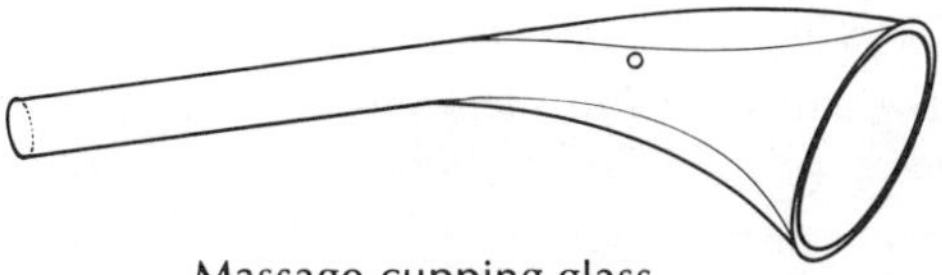

Massage cupping glass

Galvanic Apparatus

Galvanic or direct current, also known as continuous current, is the uninterrupted flow of electrons in one direction. The term *continuous* signifies that the intensity of the current is constant with respect to its magnitude and direction.

The most important effect of galvanic current is its physicochemical effect. When it passes through a chemical solution, the ions in that solution migrate in definite directions. The positive ions are attracted by the negative and vice versa.

In esthetics, the current is administered via electrodes—the anode (+) and the cathode (—) —that are connected to the two poles of a generator by flexible, insulated wires. There are always two electrodes, one to conduct the current to the person and the other to return it to the generator.

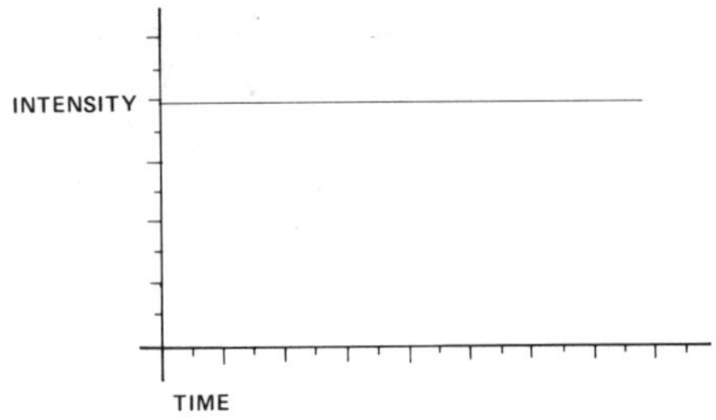

Effects of the Positive Pole	Effects of the Negative Pole
Anode (+)	Cathode (–)
Acidic reaction	Alkaline reaction
Vasoconstrictor	Vasodilator
Contraction of ostia and glands	Dilation of ostia and glands
Attracts oxygen	Attracts hydrogen
Sedative effect	Stimulant effect
Germicidal effect	
Decongestant effect	
Repels positive ions to the opposite pole	Repels negative ions to the opposite pole
Attracts negative ions	Attracts positive ions

Disincrustation. The purpose of disincrustation is to clean the skin by emulsifying or softening the excess oil (sebum) found in the skin. The ostia are frequently blocked by comedones (blackheads), accumulations of sebum and dirt that plug the opening of the sebaceous gland and prevent the gland from functioning properly.

Sebum is a waxy ester substance with a high melting point, and therefore, it is very hard. It is, however, possible to soften the sebum by saponifying it with sodium ions (Na^+). This technique consists of exposing the surface of the skin next to the comedones to a certain concentration of Na^+ ions.

Understanding the Phenomenon of Disincrustation. We have seen in an earlier chapter that the electrons of the outer orbit of an atom participate in chemical reactions when atoms combine with each other. These reactions can occur in different ways. For example, a chlorine atom normally contains 17 protons (positive) and 17 electrons (negative), thus it is electrically neutral. We also know that a sodium atom in its natural state possesses 11 negative charges (electrons) and an equal number of positive charges (protons). Regardless of the fact that both are electrically neutral, if we put a sodium atom in the presence of a chlorine atom, the following reaction will occur.

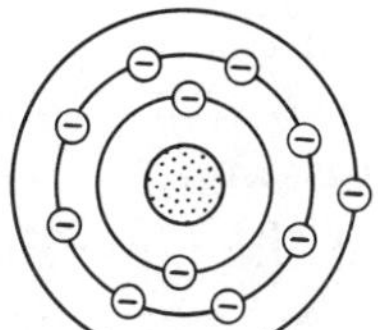

SODIUM ATOM

The sodium atom (Na) contains only a single electron in its third orbit and it tends to want to shed that electron.

By contrast, the chlorine atom (Cl) wants to complete its third orbit where it is missing a single electron. (In all atoms, a completed or saturated first orbit contains 2 electrons, while the second and third orbits always contain 8 electrons when saturated.)

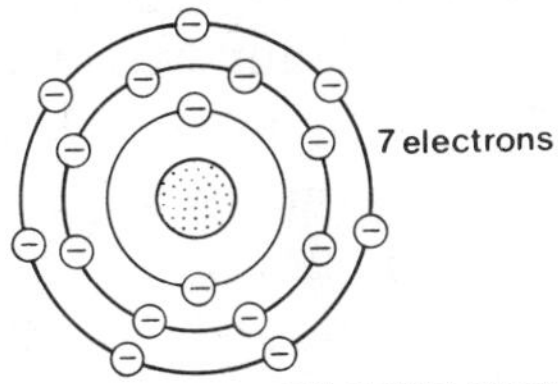

CHLORINE ATOM

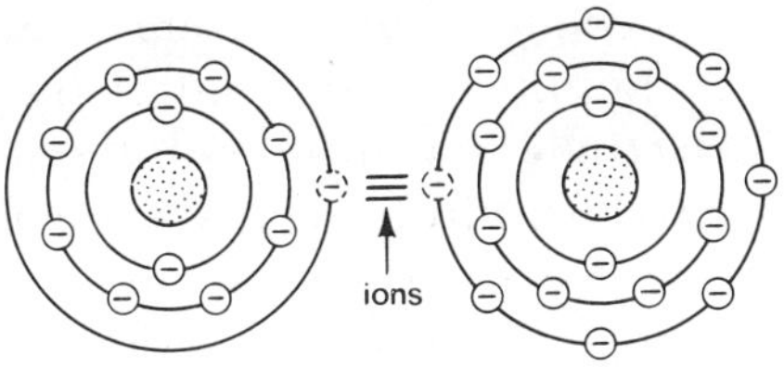

With respect to the permeability of its tissues to a galvanic current, the human body can be considered as a series of small saltwater lakes, separated by very thin cytoplasmic partitions. When molecules (such as Na^+Cl^-) are dissolved in water, they dissociate into positively charged sodium ions (Na^+) and negatively charged chloride ions (Cl^-). The flow of a direct current through the organism (saltwater) causes the ions present to migrate in definite directions. The sodium ions begin to accumulate on the contact of the active, negatively charged electrode (cathode) and the chloride ions are drawn toward the inactive (or silent), positively charged electrode (anode). The effect produced is called saponification (the reaction of a basic substance on an ester). This very reaction is what occurs in disincrustation.

How to Conduct Disincrustation. First, ask the client to remove all of her jewelry. Make certain that the switch on the galvanic apparatus is in the OFF position.

Connect the silent electrode to the positive pole (+) of the apparatus, cover it with a well-moistened spontex (or lamella), and place it in one of the client's hands.

Connect the active electrode to the negative pole (—) of the apparatus. This small electrode, a few centimeters in diameter, is covered with a layer of cotton wadding soaked in tap water containing mineral salts, the lotion used for disincrustation, or slightly salty distilled water. Turn the switch to the ON position.

Place the active electrode (—) on the client's face (which has been thoroughly cleansed) and hold it there. Gradually increase the intensity of the current using the regulator knob while checking the milliammeter. The maximum intensity to be used is that which is well tolerated by the client with no disagreeable sensations. On the average, the tolerance of the skin is in the range of 0.5 mA to 2 mA.

Move the active electrode slowly over the face *without losing contact with the skin,* concentrating on those areas with numerous comedones. The duration of the treatment must not exceed 10 to 15 minutes. At the end of the treatment while still keeping the electrode in contact with the skin, reduce the current to zero and only then lift the active electrode off the client's face.

Next, take the silent electrode from the client's hand, and lastly, turn the switch to the OFF position.

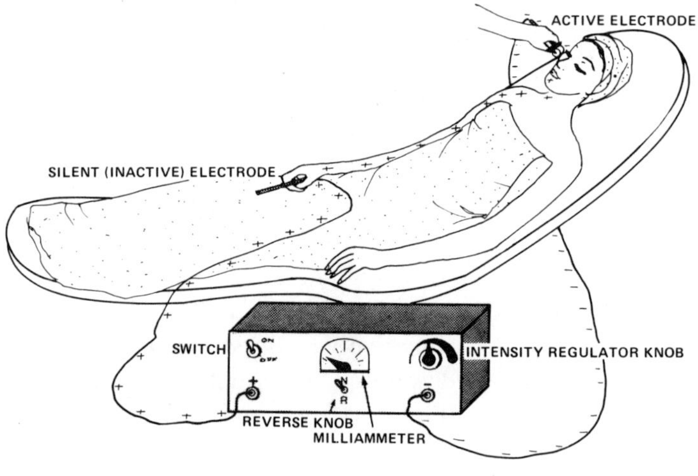

Precautions. Make certain that there are no small abrasions, cuts, pimples, and so forth, or if there are such lesions, isolate them with a bit of cream and gauze. During treatment, be sure to avoid them because a sudden change in the intensity of the current may be painful for the client. Watch the milliammeter throughout the treatment and always maintain contact with the skin of the client when there is current in the electrodes.

Disincrustation is a treatment only for occasional use and should be reserved for greasy, oily skin with multiple comedones. The technique is never to be used on sensitive or delicate skin. *Never use a galvanic current on a pregnant woman.*

Note. Never add sodium carbonate to the water used for moistening the spontex and cotton wadding. This would be a mistake because the sodium ions (Na^+) dissociated from the sodium carbonate would be attracted to the negatively charged active electrode where they would collect and repel the ions of the skin and comedones. The saponification reaction would thus be neutralized and no disincrustation would take place. Moreover, if the skin comes in contact with a strongly alkaline solution, such as sodium carbonate, it becomes irritated and the pH will be modified.

Disincrustation Using Oranges. Disincrustation using oranges is to be used for oily skin and poor complexions.

Press the tips of each of the leads coming from the positive and negative poles of the apparatus into a half of an orange. Place one of the halves on each side of the client's face. Slowly increase the intensity of the current using the regulator knob. Gently slide the orange halves over the face and neck for two or three minutes.

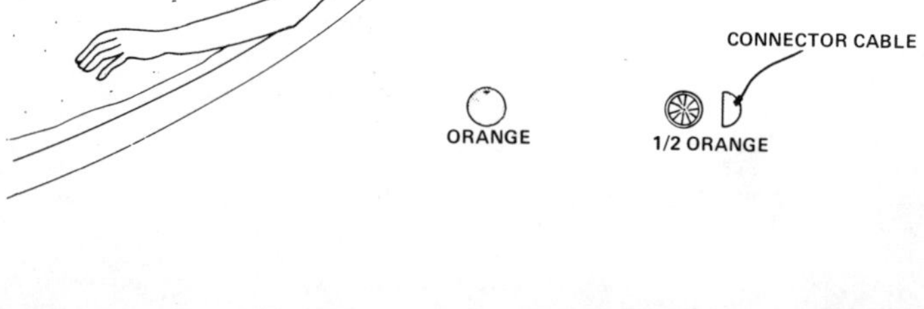

Lower the intensity, reverse the current, and repeat the same process for another two or three minutes.

After the treatment, rinse the face well with warm water, followed by a warm atomization, and then continue with the remainder of the treatment.

Ionization. The purpose of ionization is to facilitate the penetration of certain active products into the skin. The theory of ionization hardly differs from that of disincrustation. When a product is ionized by an electric current, it can penetrate in the form of dissociated ions. Thus, it is necessary to use ionizable substances with a known polarity. The polarity of the active electrode is adjusted according to the polarity of the ionizable substance employed.

Procedure. After a thorough cleansing, the selected product is applied to the client's face. If the ionizable product is positive (+), the active electrode is attached to the positive pole (+) of the apparatus, and the inactive (silent) electrode to the negative pole (—) of the apparatus. If the ionizable product is negative (—), the electrodes are connected in the reverse manner.

Use the same procedure as for disincrustation and observe the same precautions. Never ionize products on sensitive or irritated skin, and never use the technique with a pregnant woman.

Mask Method. A mask is usually made of spontex and has two openings or pockets, one on each side, in which the small

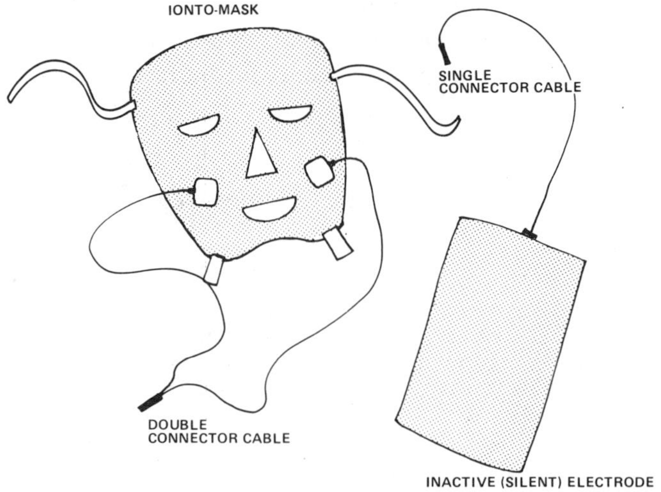

plates or active electrodes may be inserted. The serum or ionizable product is applied to the client's face, and then a tissue or a well-moistened special paper mask is placed over the face. The ionto mask, once it has been well moistened, is then placed on the face over the paper. The mask must be placed appropriately on the face and tied on behind the head.

The inactive electrode is a rather large metal plate, enclosed in a layer of damp spontex. It is placed either under the back, near the neck, or on one arm, attached by an elastic band.

Method Using a Cataphoresis Roller. The cataphoresis roller is used for treating large surfaces, such as the face, neck, and décolleté. It is also used when it is necessary to avoid certain areas or when the client suffers from claustrophobia.

The metal roller is enclosed in a thin layer of well-moistened cotton wadding. The ionizable preparation is applied to the client's skin. The roller becomes the active electrode, and its polarity is adjusted according to that of the ionizable product; the inactive electrode is either a manual electrode that has been covered with a lamella or damp spontex or a metal plate covered with a damp spontex.

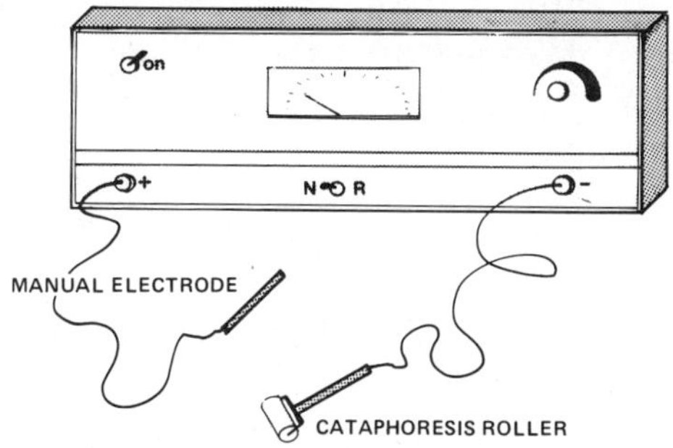

Derivative Method. The derivative method can be used for products that are positively and negatively ionized. For example, amino acid molecules and certain tissular placental extracts possess the peculiar characteristic of having two ions of opposite charge attached to the core of the molecule at the same time. These substances are all very complex chemically, each molecule often being comprised of dozens of atoms. The molecules do not simply dissociate as do the two-atom salts described above.

Rather, if we place such a molecule in an electric current, it will first align itself so that its positive portion (+) is oriented toward the negative pole (—) and the negative portion (—) is oriented toward the positive pole (+). Then it will become displaced or distorted, according to the polar attractions, toward a point situated somewhere between the two poles. The displacement ceases at the point of equilibrium called the "isoelectric point." This point is specific for each amino acid and can be used for identification purposes.

This method can only be employed with substances that simultaneously form two ions on the same molecule. With all other substances, the second phase of this technique would destroy everything that had been obtained in the first phase.

The ionizable product is applied to the face of the client. Then, two metal plates covered with moist spontex are placed one beside the other under the client's back near the nape of the neck. One of the plates is connected to the positive pole (+) of the apparatus and the other to the negative pole (—). The current should be reversed midway through the treatment, for example, three minutes positive (+) and three minutes negative (—). Massage manipulations may be performed during treatment.

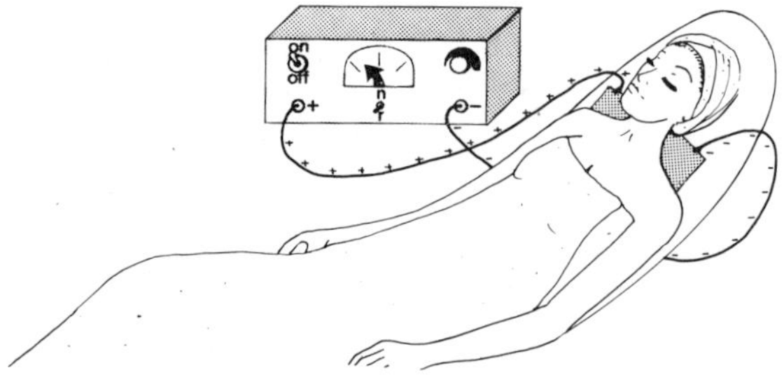

Ionizing Galvanic Douche

It is possible to perform a galvanic douche by utilizing the galvanic apparatus and the cold atomizer at the same time.

Place the tip of one of the two leads in one of the two outlets on the galvanic apparatus; using a metal clamp (alligator clip) attach the other end of the same wire to the stream sprayer of the cold atomizer. The manual electrode, wrapped in a wet spontex or lamella, is connected to the other pole of the galvanic apparatus and given to the client to hold. The spray therefore becomes the active electrode and the manual electrode becomes the inactive or silent electrode.

The esthetician must be careful to use salinated water or a lotion containing agents that conduct electricity, for example, salicylic acid mixed in a lotion. For the treatment of acne, a camphorated lotion is used.

Purpose

Cleansing and disincrustation of hard-to-reach areas (edges around the nose) .

Treatment of seborrhea or acne. (The active electrode is connected to the positive pole of the galvanic apparatus in order to provide an acidic reaction.)

Treatment of superficial dehydration using a moisturizing lotion.

Procedure. Plug in the two instruments to an electrical outlet, and connect them using an alligator clip. Seat the client and have her hold the face pan with one hand and the inactive elec-

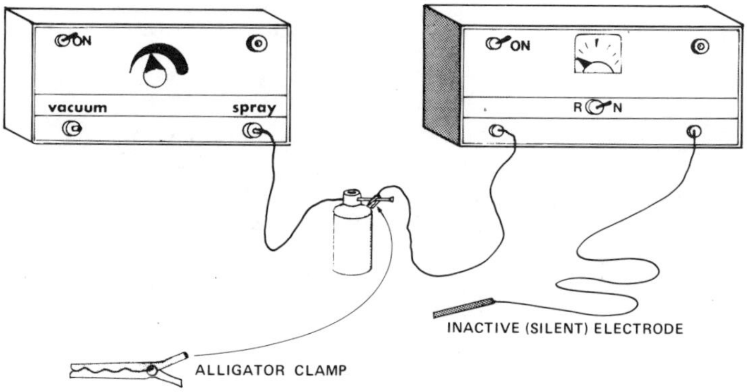

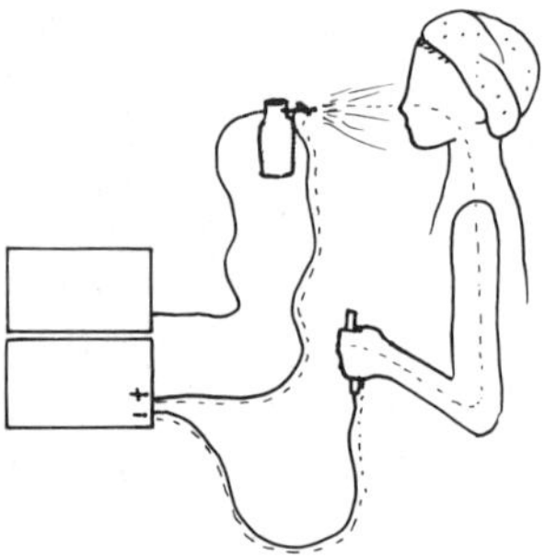

trode with the other. Fill the container with salinated water or an appropriate lotion. Direct the spray toward the client's face, and turn the switches of both instruments to the ON position. With the thumb, close the opening at the top of the cap so that the spray can start. Slowly increase the intensity of the galvanic apparatus up to about 2 mA, and atomize the areas to be treated for about ten minutes. Reduce the intensity of the current to zero, and remove the thumb from the top of the cannister to stop the spray. Sponge off the client's face well, and proceed with the rest of the treatment.

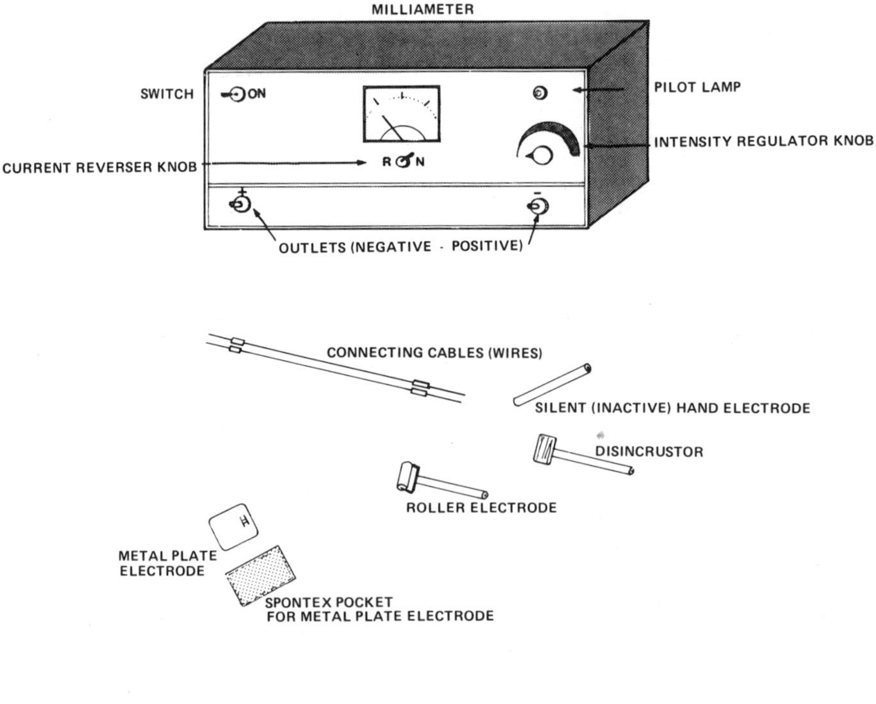

Directions for use. Before turning on the apparatus, place one end of the red wire in the red outlet of the apparatus [positive pole (+)], and attach the electrode to the other end of the wire. Then, place one end of the black wire in the black outlet of the apparatus [negative pole (—)], and attach the other end to the second electrode. Depending on the treatment to be performed, the positive or negative electrode will become the active electrode. Check the reverse knob; at the N (normal) position, the polarity of the electrodes conforms to the poles of the apparatus where they are attached. Turn the switch to the ON position.

Have the client hold the inactive (silent) electrode in her hand and put the active electrode on her face. While moving the active electrode, increase the intensity very slowly to the desired level, always taking the client's degree of sensitivity into consideration. At the end of the treatment, reduce the intensity to the minimum before removing the electrodes. Turn off the switch.

Polarity Test

1. Attach the two conducting wires to the two poles of the galvanic apparatus, and put the other ends of the wires into a container of slightly salinated water. Take care that the two wires remain at least two inches apart. Increase the intensity of the current to the maximum level. As soon as the current passes through, a large number of bubbles will collect around the tip of the wire connected to the negative pole.
2. Moisten pH indicator paper with demineralized water. Attach the two conducting wires to the two poles of the galvanic apparatus and raise the intensity to the maximum level. Press the other ends of the wires into the pH indicator paper. The wire attached to the negative pole will turn the paper green (alkaline reaction).

Precautions: GALVANIC CURRENT CAN BURN THE SKIN

1. Avoid bringing the metal portion of the electrodes into contact with the client's skin.

2. Always watch the milliammeter during treatment.
3. Always maintain contact with the client's face while current is flowing through the electrodes.

12

Products Used in Esthetics

THE BASIC COMPOSITION OF A COSMETIC

A list giving the basic composition of a cosmetic follows.

Essential Component:	Example: Lanolin
Active Ingredient:	Example: Azulene

Preservative: Example: Tegosept M (methyl paraben)

Antioxidant: Example: Vitamin C (ascorbic acid)

Perfume: Example: Essential oils (lemon, eucalyptus, and so forth)

CLASSIFICATION AND DESCRIPTION OF DIFFERENT TYPES OF PRODUCTS

Emulsions: A mixture of oil and water made miscible through the use of a third ingredient called an *emulsifier.* There are three types of emulsions: Oil in water (O/W), water in oil (W/O), and dual emulsions.

Description of an oil in water emulsion: Is evanescent, aqueous and hydroscopic; it mixes with water, is slightly acidic, is a good moisturizer and conductor of electricity.

Description of a water in oil emulsion: Forms an ointment or salve which is oily and hydrophobic; it cannot be diluted by water and usually has a slightly alkaline pH; it soothes and lubricates the skin but does not conduct electricity.

Description of a dual emulsion: Is intermediate between aqueous and oily (e.g., creams made from a mixture of beeswax and borax).

Suspensions: Suspensions are composed of solid particles that float in a liquid without dissolving. (They must be shaken well before use.)

Soaps (cake): Usually presented in the form of rectangular bars, which come in a paper wrapping or sometimes a box.

Soaps: Ordinary soap is alkaline with a pH usually in the range of 8.5 to 11. It cleans as a result of the action of a base (soda, potash) on fatty acids (lard, and so forth).

Cakes: A cake has an acidic pH in the range of 4 to 6. It hardly lathers at all. Some cakes have a neutral pH (7). Occasionally, glycerine or lanolin is added.

Note: Detergent is a synthetic soap and possesses the same properties except that sometimes it is not alkaline. Most washing creams are detergents and normally have an acidic pH.

Lotions or Aromatic Waters: Aqueous solutions, composed of essential oils and distilled water, are very often colored. Some contain 5 to 20 percent alcohol.

Powders: Solids that have been pulverized into very tiny particles; they are composed of talc, zinc oxide, amidon, and so forth, and are often perfumed.

Pastes: Substances whose thickness can be increased or decreased according to the amount of powder added to the base (emulsion). Used to treat only the surface of the horny layer. Some pastes, which are prepared in advance like masks, can be diluted with demineralized water or a lotion.

Oils: Substances formed primarily of fatty acids and amino vegetable bases (e.g., avocado oil), animal bases (e.g., turtle oil), or mineral bases. They usually serve as the base of an emulsion. Lipids, fixed oils, and fats are all oils. *Note:* Not to be confused with essential or volatile oils (e.g., rose essence), which are obtained by distilling aromatic vegetable substances.

Gels: Colloidal, semisolid dispersions that are usually moisturizing; they often contain alcohol and penetrate the skin very well; most are cooling and are conductors of electricity.

Masks: Preparations to be applied to the face; they come in different forms: creams, powders, pastes, gels. Their action depends on the active ingredients they contain.

PURPOSES OF THE DIFFERENT PRODUCTS USED IN ESTHETICS

Cleansing Milks (Emulsions)

Clean the surface of the skin by emulsifying the secretions (oils), dirt, makeup, powder, and so forth. They must have a neutral pH or be just slightly acidic, depending on the type of skin.

Cleansing Creams (Cold Cream Type, Emulsions)

Clean the surface of the skin by emulsifying oils, makeup, powder but leave a greasy film on the skin. They are particularly useful for removing theatrical makeup or very thick makeup.

Note. After use, the skin should be cleansed to remove the greasy film left by the cleansing cream.

Washing Creams (Emulsions, Pastes, Cakes)

Most washing creams have a slightly acidic pH. They can be used at the institute for a thorough cleansing after a milk and lotion.

The lather can be worked up by moving the fingertips in a circular motion on the face or with a complexion brush.

They can also be used at home instead of the milks for removing makeup (in the presence of acne, comedones, and so forth) or once or twice a week for a good cleansing before using a serum.

Note. Washing creams that have had enzymes (e.g., almond bran) or granules (e.g., sea sand) added possess the additional effects of oxygenating and brightening the skin.

Neutral Cakes, Acidic Cakes

Neutral cakes (pH 7) can be used to cleanse normal young skin. Acidic cakes, which generally have a pH of 4 to 5, are primarily used for acne conditions and oily skin.

Note. Protracted use of an overly acidic preparation dehydrates the skin.

Lotions or Aromatic Waters (Solutions)

These products are used following a cleansing milk in order to complete the cleansing by removing the residual oily film and dirt that might still be present on the skin. The action of the lotion varies according to which essence was used and the percentage of alcohol in the solution: calming (linden), soothing (rose), mild decongestant (witch hazel), astringent (briar), and so forth.

Note. Be cautious with lotions containing alcohol because they dry, dehydrate, and irritate the skin.

Mild Peelings or Lysings, Controlled Peelings (Powders, Crystals)

Made primarily from proteolytic enzymes (digestive enzymes that split, dissolve or digest any nonliving matter), usually papain, trypsin, pepsin.

By penetrating into the ostia of the skin, they can liquify the sebum, reduce color spots, brighten the complexion, refine the skin, and improve its respiration. These "peelings" never attack living skin cells. On the contrary, they digest the dead cells of the superficial layers of the epidermis. They must be used at the institute under the supervision of an esthetician. There is no danger of harm and they are ideal for use as deep cleansers. They are particularly recommended for the care of asphyxic skin and before starting treatment with serums.

Note. Always carefully follow the directions provided for use and moisturize the skin well at the end of treatment.

Gumming Masks (Pastes)

Include mechanical peelings, rubbings, and gum treatments. A light mask layer is to be applied to the face and allowed to dry. By gumming with the fingers, the dead cells from the epidermis are eliminated.

Note. Some masks contain enzymes, such as papain, and thus come under the heading of lysings.

Serums (Emulsions, Solutions, Oils)

Serums are concentrated products containing active ingredients in their pure state, sealed in sterile ampuls, and presented in different forms (aqueous, oily). Their effects vary according to their active ingredients: nourishing (e.g., embryonic extracts), antiseptic (e.g., yeast), softening, soothing (e.g., azulene). These are the most effective products in esthetics, and thus they must always be used on well-prepared skin so that they can penetrate into the deep tissues.

Note. Any opened ampul must be used immediately because the serum deteriorates upon contact with air or with any unsterilized object.

Masks (Pastes, Emulsions, Gels, Powders)

Products to be applied and left on the face and neck until dry (about 15 or 20 minutes). Their effects vary according to their active ingredients. Some can act as skin bracers, others can reduce redness, brighten the complexion or help serums penetrate more fully. The principle effect of a mask, however, is to relax the features of the face.

Note. An aqueous serum must never be applied before, but always after, a mud mask composed of kaolin or argile (clay).

Protective Creams or Day Creams (Emulsions)

These products are moisturizing creams that leave a thin film on the skin. This film acts to protect the skin against dirt and pollution. It also prevents powder and makeup base from obstructing the ostia.

Note. Protective or day creams must be used every day in the morning after a thorough cleansing.

Treatment Creams or Night Creams (Emulsions)

These creams contain such active ingredients as placentary or embryonic extracts, royal jelly, and collagen, and their purpose is to nourish the skin. They must be applied in the evening to the face and neck following a light cleansing.

Note. It is always preferable to apply these creams about 30 minutes before going to bed so that they have time to penetrate completely.

Sun Filters (Emulsions, Lotions, Jellies, Oils)

These products contain substances capable of obstructing most harmful rays of the sun while still allowing the rays for tanning to pass through to the skin.

PRINCIPAL VEGETABLE SUBSTANCES USED IN THE MANUFACTURE OF COSMETICS

It is important to realize that there are no natural cosmetics, as such, but that the ingredients of cosmetics are sometimes extracted from natural sources. Sometimes a particular ingredient that is found in nature can also be made chemically or artificially. Regardless, the effect is the same because the ingredient is chemically the same.

When manufacturing cosmetics, it is necessary to add moisturizers, oils, one or two emulsifiers, a preservative, an antioxidant, an antiseptic, and, sometimes, a perfume to the basic ingredients.

Among the various vegetable substances used in cosmetics, are extracts from fruits and vegetables and even the leaves, bark, and roots of certain trees and plants. Just as fruits and vegetables are important in our daily diet, they are important for the health of the skin. Beautiful skin depends on a person's general state of health as well as on the external care given it.

The following table gives a general idea of the principal components of various vegetable substances, their effects on the skin, their uses—either in their natural state in lotions, infusions, decoctions or as ingredients added to creams, ointments, and masks.

Principal Components of Vegetable Substances—Their Effect on the Skin

Name	Main Components	General Effects	Recommended For
ABSINTH	Essential oils, iron, tannin	Astringent, cicatrizant, diuretic	Oily skins, large pores, acneic skins
AGRIMONY	Essence Tannin	Astringent, anti-inflammatory	Oily skins, large pores, acneic skins
ALGAE	Numerous minerals, iodine, multivitamin complexes, glucides, several amino acids	Nutrient mineral supplement, moisturizer, tonic	All skins; aging, deficient, and dehydrated skins
ALMOND	Starch, oil, glucides, vitamins A and B, calcium	Nutrient, lubricant, soothing	Alipoidic skins, dehydrated skins

Principal Components of Vegetable Substances—Their Effect on the Skin (*continued*)

Name	Main Components	General Effects	Recommended For
ALOE	Resin, amino acids, glucides	Cicatrizant, tonic, nutrient	Aging skins, dehydrated skins
ANGELICA	Tannin, malic acid, resin	Calming, tonic, astringent, aromatic	Discolored skins, atonic skins
APPLE	Phosphorus, calcium, copper, sodium, magnesium, iron, potassium, glucides, malic acid	Antiseptic, disinfectant, firming, brightens complexion, astringent	Oily skins, atonic skins, blotchy complexions and skin eruptions
APRICOT	Essential oils, vitamin A, mineral salts	Regenerating the skin, nutrient	Normal skins
ARNICA	Camphor, malic acid, fat substances	Relieves congestion, antiseptic, soothing	Sensitive skins, blotchy skins, oily and acneic skins
ARTICHOKE	Mineral salts, proteins, vitamin B	Diuretic, tonic, tissue rejuvenating, depurative, brightens complexion	Aging skins, asphyxic skins, pigment spots, reduces fat accumulations (cellulitis)
BANANA	Oils, starch, iron, glucides, lime, vitamins A, B, C, E	Nutrient, moisturizer	Alipoidic skins, dehydrated skins
BILBERRY	Tannin, glucides, organic acids	Astringent, cicatrizant, tonic	Oily skins, large pores, atonic skins
BIRCH	Tannin, aromatic essence, phosphorus, sodium, resin	Depurative, calming	Dehydrated skins, various skin rashes (dartre), erythema, chapping, dermatosis
BLACKBERRY	Tannin, malic acid, organic acids, lime, iron, sodium	Astringent, diuretic	Oily skins, large pores
BLACK CURRANT	Malic acid, vitamin C	Diuretic, anti-inflammatory, relieves congestion, refreshing	Sensitive skins, blotchy skins
BLUEBERRY	Tannin, natural methyl salicylate	Astringent, soothing, antiinflammatory	Sensitive skins, blotchy skins, relieves congestion; used mainly around the eyes

Principal Components of Vegetable Substances—Their Effect on the Skin (*continued*)

Name	Main Components	General Effects	Recommended For
BURDOCK	Essential oils, tannin, potassium, lime, magnesium, inulin	Depurative, astringent, cicatrizant, disinfectant	Seborrheic skins, acneic skins, eczema, scalp treatment (against hair falling out)
CABBAGE	Sulphur, iron, iodine, glucides, lime, vitamins A and D	Cicatrizant, disinfectant	Acneic skins, boils
CACTUS	Mineral salts	Calming, tonic	Sensitive skins, dehydrated skins
CAMOMILE	Lime, potassium, phosphorus, azulene	Calming, tonic, antiseptic	Sensitive skins, inflamed skins, dehydrated skins, sunburns; mild bleaching of the hair
CAMPHOR TREE	Raw camphor	Antiseptic	Acneic skins
CARROT	Vitamin A (carotene), glucides, iron, iodine, potassium, magnesium, lime	Moisturizer, regenerating	Dehydrated skins, sensitive skins, pilary keratosis, various skin rashes (dartre)
CELERY	Proteins, vitamins A, B, C	Depurative, refreshing	All skins
CHERVIL	Oil, palmetic acid	Nutrient, regenerating	All skins
CHESTNUT	Tannin, glucides, starch, lipids, proteins	Astringent, nutrient, calming	All skins, aging skins, wrinkles
COMMON COMFREY	Tannin, mucilage, allantoin, essential oils	Astringent, soothing, cicatrizant, moisturizer, emollient	Dehydrated skins, acneic skins, sunburns, erythema, chapping
CUCUMBER	Glucides, starch, vitamins A, B, C	Diuretic, refreshing, soothing, slightly astringent	All skins, reduces fat accumulation (cellulitis)
DANDELION	Iron, phosphorus, potassium, sodium, latex	Diuretic, depurative, tonic, regenerating	All skins, cellulitis treatment
DOG'S GRASS	Potassium, glucides, mucilage	Diuretic, emollient, refreshing	All skins
EGGPLANT	Proteins, vitamins A, C	Moisturizer, regenerating	Aging skins, dehydrated skins
ELDER TREE	Malic acid, potassium, iron, glucides, mucilage, organic acid	Diuretic, soothing, emollient	Sensitive skins, inflamed skins, dehydrated and alipoidic skins, various skin rashes

Principal Components of Vegetable Substances—Their Effect on the Skin (*continued*)

Name	Main Components	General Effects	Recommended For
FENNEL	Iron, potassium, lime, sulphur, phosphorus, essence	Vasoconstrictor, tonic, relieves congestion, regenerating	Aging skins, discolored skins, blotchy skins
FIG TREE	Glucides, oil, proteins, vitamin C, resin	Moisturizer, emollient, regenerating	Dehydrated skins, various skin rashes (dartre)
GENTIAN	Glucides, pectin (enzyme), oils, mucilage, essence	Tonic, depurative, soothing	Wrinkled skins, atonic skins
GERMAN CAMOMILE	Azulene essence, lime, phosphorus, potassium	Antiinflammatory, cicatrizant, tonic, brightens complexion	Sensitive skins, dehydrated skins, blotchy complexions, bleaches hair
GINSENG	Starch, glucides, phytosterin, hormones	Stimulating, revitalizing, soothing, regenerating, improves circulation	Aging skins, wrinkles, atonic skins, blotchy skins
GOURD	Proteins, vitamins A, B, C	Regenerating, cicatrizant, moisturizer	All skins
GRAPEFRUIT	Citric acid, glucides, vitamins A, C	Astringent, brightens complexion	Oily skins, large pores, blotchy complexions
GRAPES	Sodium, glucides, vitamins A, B_2, E	Diuretic, depurative, regenerating, cicatrizant	Acneic skins, comedo-prone skins
HOP PLANT	Tannin, essential oils, resin, hormones	Tonic, depurative, astringent, regenerating	Aging skins, large pores
HORSE CHESTNUTS	Fat oils, starch, tannin, vitamin P, saponin	Venous tonic, vasoconstrictor, relieves congestion	Blotchy skins, aging skins, varicose veins
IRIS	Tannin, starch	Diuretic, depurative, astringent, soothing	Oily skins, inflamed skins
IVY	Tannin, hormones (estrogen)	Vasoconstrictor, reduces congestion, emollient, firming, calming	Atonic skins, reduces fat accumulation (cellulitis), inflamed skins
LAVENDER	Essence, oils	Antiseptic, disinfectant, calming	Acneic skins, eczema, burns (sunburns)
LEEK	Glucides, sulphur, vitamins B, C, alkaline salts	Antiseptic, calming, reinforces capillaries	Blotchy skins, inflamed skins, burns, sunburns

Principal Components of Vegetable Substances—Their Effect on the Skin (*continued*)

Name	Main Components	General Effects	Recommended For
LEMON PLANT	Essential oils, iron, potassium, tannin	Astringent, muscular firming, vasoconstrictor	All skins, atonic skins
LEMON	Citric acid, glucides, vitamins C, B, P	Disinfectant, antiseptic, astringent, brightens complexion	Oily skins, large pores, blotchy and discolored complexions
LETTUCE	Proteins, vitamins A, B, C, glucides, chlorophyll, mineral salts	Diuretic, calming, emollient	Inflamed skins, dehydrated skins
LILY	Iron, oils	Emollient, calming, soothing	Sensitive skins, dehydrated skins, inflamed skins, burns, sunburns
LINDEN TREE	Essence, tannin, glucides, sterols, vitamin C, iron, lime	Calming, emollient, sudorific	Sensitive skins, inflamed skins, all skins
MALLOW	Mucilage, lime, iron, potassium, sodium, sulphur	Calming, emollient	Inflamed skins, all skins
MANDARIN (TANGERINE)	Citric acid, malic acid, mineral salts, vitamins A, B, C, P	Tonic, astringent, regenerating	Oily skins, large pores
MARIGOLD	Essential oils, salicylic acid, mucilage, sulphur, phosphorus	Depurative, diuretic, antiseptic, cicatrizant, reinforces capillaries	Acneic skins, various skin rashes (dartre), eczema, furunculosis, inflamed skins, burns, sunburns
MARSH-MALLOW	Mucilage, fine oils, starch, glucides, lime, iron, potassium, sodium, sulphur	Soothing, emollient, antiinflammatory, cicatrizant	Inflamed skins, acneic skins, boils, various skin rashes (dartre), chapping
MINT	Tannin, menthol essence, oil, iron	Antiseptic, calming, increases permeability of the capillaries, astringent	Oily skins, acneic skins, large pores, blotchy skins
MULBERRY	Malic acid, lactic acid, methyl salicylate, tannin, pectin	Astringent, cicatrizant, analgesic, diuretic	Acneic skins, large pores
NASTURTIUM	Sulphurated essence, benzyl essence	Diuretic, stimulating	Scalp treatment to prevent hair falling out

Principal Components of Vegetable Substances—Their Effect on the Skin (*continued*)

Name	Main Components	General Effects	Recommended For
NETTLE	Tannin, chlorophyll, iron, sulphur, silica, calcium, mucilage, potassium, vitamin A	Tonic, astringent, depurative, diuretic, vasoconstrictor, antiseptic	Acneic skins, oily skins, large pores, eczema, scalp treatment
OATS	Albumin, fat, nitrate, potassium, phosphorus, nitrogen, lime	Moisturizing, nutrient	Alipoidic skins, dehydrated skins
ORANGE	Essential oils, citric acid, vitamins A, C	Astringent, refreshing, brightens complexion	Normal skins, oily skins, large pores, blotchy complexions
ORCHID	Mucilage, starch, lime, phosphorus, sodium	Stimulating, moisturizing	All skins
PARSLEY	Oil, palmetic acid, proteins, vitamins A, C, chlorophyll	Diuretic, improves blood circulation, relieves congestion, stimulating	All skins, inflamed skins, blotchy skins, fatigued skins
PEACH	Essential oils, glucides, vitamins A, C	Calming, soothing, diuretic	All skins
PEAR	Glucides, tannin, vitamins A, B, P	Depurative, diuretic, emollient, soothing	Sensitive skins, inflamed skins
PLANTAIN	Tannin, sulphur, alkaline salts, lime, potassium, vitamins A, C, E	Astringent, cicatrizant, depurative, emollient	Acneic skins, large pores
POTATO	Iron, potassium, proteins, glucides, starch, vitamin C	Tonic, nutrient	Aging skins, atonic skins, water retention (aqueous bags mainly under the eyes)
RASPBERRY	Tannin, citric acid, malic acid, lime, sodium	Diuretic, depurative, astringent, refreshing, strengthening	Oily skins, large pores
RED CURRANT	Potassium, lime, malic acid, citric acid, glucides, vitamins A, B, C	Diuretic, astringent, calming	Oily skins, large pores
RHUBARB	Malic acid, oxalic acid, lime, iron, glucides	Astringent, diuretic tonic	Faded skins, aging skins, large pores
ROSE	Essential oils, tannin	Astringent, anti-inflammatory, tonic, soothing	All skins; also for compresses on eyelids

Principal Components of Vegetable Substances—Their Effect on the Skin (*continued*)

Name	Main Components	General Effects	Recommended For
SAGE	Tannin, potassium essence, lime	Stimulating, tonic, anti-sudorific	All skins, atonic skins
SEAWEED	Essential oils, mucilage, vitamins B_1, C, E, iodine, iron	Reduces fatty tissues, activates blood circulation, dissolves fat accumulation	Aging skins, mostly for cellulitis treatment
SOYA BEAN	Proteins, oil, lecithin, amino acids, phosphorus, nitrogen, vitamins A, B, E	Emulsifier, moisturizer, nutrient	Alipoidic skins, dehydrated skins
SORREL	Iron, potassium, oxalic acid	Diuretic, depurative, revitalizing, astringent	All skins
SPINACH	Proteins, iron, mucilage, vitamins A, B, C	Soothing, regenerating, reinforces capillaries, moisturizes	Dehydrated skins, aging skins, blotchy skins
SAINT-JOHN'S-WORT	Essential oils, tannin, coloring substances (pigment)	Antiseptic, astringent, diuretic, calming	Acneic skins, inflamed skins, burns, sunburns
STRAWBERRY	Tannin, salicylic acid, iron, lime, sodium	Astringent, diuretic, depurative, refreshing, firming	Oily skins, blotchy complexions
SUNFLOWER	Glucides, oil, starch	Emollient, moisturizer	All skins
THYME	Essence, thymol, aromatic oils, camphor	Stimulating, strengthening, anti-septic, antibacterial	Acneic skins, infections of the skin
TOMATO	Malic acid, glucides, vitamins A, B, C	Emollient, brightens complexion, increases skin's acidity	Blotchy complexions, alkaline-prone skins, oily skins, comedoes
TORMENTIL	Tannin, oil, iron	Astringent	Large pores
TURNIP	Vitamins B, C, glucides, sulphur, mineral salts	Vasoconstrictor, acts on the skin's capillaries, regenerating, cicatrizant	Blotchy skins, dehydrated skins, acneic skins, boils
VALERIAN	Essence, glucides, malic acid	Calming	All skins, treatment of the scalp
VIOLET	Salicylic acid, oil, essence, mucilage	Emollient, diuretic, sudorific	All skins, slightly dehydrated skins

Principal Components of Vegetable Substances—Their Effect on the Skin (*continued*)

Name	Main Components	General Effects	Recommended For
WALNUT	Tannin, oil, vitamin C, iron, potassium, sulphur, malic acid, vegetable albumin	Tonic, astringent, depurative, antiseptic	All skins; some ointments and creams used for the treatment of certain types of dermatoses are made from walnut leaves
WATERCRESS	Sulphur, iron, iodine, vitamin C, glucides	Diuretic, stimulant, emollient, depurative	Dermatosis, pigment spots, chapping; scalp treatment to prevent hair falling out
WATERLILY	Mucilage, starch, oil, hormones	Moisturizer, nutrient, regenerating	All skins
WHEAT	Proteins, starch, potassium hydroxide, vitamins A, B, PP, albumin	Regenerating, nutrient	Dehydrated skins, alipoidic skins, aging skins
WHEATGERM	Vitamin B (niacin), proteins, iron	Antiinflammatory, emollient, soothing, calming, regenerating	Sensitive skins, dehydrated skins, inflamed skins
WILLOW	Tannin, glucides, salicyclic acid, hormones	Antiseptic, astringent, tonic	All skins, acneic skins, comedo-prone skins
WINTER CHERRY	Citric acid, vitamin C	Diuretic, depurative, calming, emollient	All skins, sensitive skins, dehydrated skins
WITCH HAZEL	Tannin, essential oils, lime, potassium hydroxide, iron	Vasoconstrictor, tonic, astringent; normalizes blood circulation	Blotchy skins, atonic skins, varicose veins
YEAST (BREWER'S)	Phosphorus, potassium hydroxide, magnesium, glucides, lipids, proteins, enzymes, vitamin B complex	Tonic, stimulant, accelerates chemical reactions, regenerating	Acneic skins, dermatosis, asphyxic and comedo-prone skins

13

Treatments and Advice for the Client

This chapter will contain step by step descriptions of a typical treatment and of various specific treatments for different types of skin and skin conditions.

Each specific treatment will also contain several recommendations for the customers so that the salon treatment may be continued at home for better and faster results.

TYPICAL TREATMENT (SUGGESTED METHOD)

Light Cleansing

Wash with:

Cleansing milk

Lotion

Warm atomization

Skin Analysis

File: Perform the skin analysis and fill out the client's personal record.

Deep Cleansing

From among the various cleansing techniques below, select the most appropriate one, based on the examination of the skin:

Galvanic disincrustation
Galvanic douche
Peeling
Lysing
Washing cream
Acidic or neutral cake
Warm mask

Finish with a second warm atomization.

Note. For the client's first visit, it is advisable to proceed to a very light cleansing, such as washing cream or other.

Warm Vaporizer

From 15 to 20 minutes

Extraction of Comedones

Use a vacuum apparatus, a comedo-extractor, or perform manually.

High Frequency

Violet or neon ray electrodes

Serums

A serum can be atomized or worked into the skin by indirect massage if it is aqueous, by manual massage if it is oily, or by ionization with the galvanic apparatus if it is ionizable.

Mask

The mask must be applied with a brush or the fingers and left on the face for approximately 15 to 20 minutes. Creamy or gel masks are normally applied after the serum. By contrast, mud masks are to be applied *before* the serum if the serum to be used is aqueous.

Imbibition

With a protective or treatment cream

Note. For the treatment of wrinkles, sagging or settling skin or for activation of circulation, manual massages can be performed or an antiwrinkle or Jacquet cupping glass can be used in conjunction with a vacuum apparatus. There is other equipment that can be used in esthetics but it will not be discussed in this book.

Advice for the Esthetician

Throughout the treatment, make every effort to be as quiet as possible, do not make needless conversation, and be discreet. Coordinate and connect massage movements without losing contact with the client. Always assume contact with the client gently so as not to startle her. Always begin treatment with a warm atomization and conclude it with a cold atomization. The esthetician must always take the condition of her client's skin and her age into consideration before starting a particular treatment or recommending products.

TREATMENT FOR NORMAL SKIN

Purpose of Treatment

To preserve the skin's freshness and radiance; to prevent dehydration and premature aging

Light Cleansing

Wash with:

Cleansing milk with a linden, apricot, or other base

Lotion with a similar base

Initial warm atomization

Skin Analysis

The client's personal file

Deep Cleansing

Select from among the following:

Acidic or neutral cake, nongranular washing cream, and so forth. This type of skin does not require more than two to four light "peelings" per year (unless changes in the skin occur) in order to preserve its freshness, help it eliminate dead cells, and facilitate nutritional exchange.

Conclude treatment with a second warm atomization.

Warm Vaporizer

Approximately 15 minutes

Extraction of Comedones

If necessary

High Frequency

Use a violet ray electrode to disinfect by sparking if comedones were extracted. Activate circulation, decongest, and relax the skin using the neon ray electrode.

Serum

Apply a moisturizing serum with a turtle oil base to prevent dehydration or any other serum suitable for the particular treatment of a temporary alteration of the skin.

Mask

Apply a moisturizing mask or any other mask, depending upon the temporary skin problem.

Imbibition

With a light moisturizing cream

Advice for the Client

Face should be thoroughly cleansed morning and evening with a cleansing milk, followed by a lotion appropriate for the skin type. A protective cream should always be used. If the client does not visit the institute regularly, recommend that she cleanse her skin well once a week with a nongranular washing cream. If necessary, also recommend a very light night (treatment) cream to be used two or three times a week. Always advise that she use a sun filter (oil or cream) before exposing her skin to the sun.

TREATMENT FOR DELICATE OR SENSITIVE SKIN

Purpose of Treatment

To preserve or reestablish suppleness

To prevent dehydration

To prevent or reduce redness

To stimulate firmness in the skin thereby preventing sagging

Note. Persons with this skin type tend to have allergies, thus gumming, disincrustation, and ionization are to be avoided.

Light Cleansing

Wash with:

Cleansing milk with an azulene base

Lotion with a hamamelis (witch hazel) base

Initial warm atomization

Skin Analysis

The client's personal file

Deep Cleansing

Select one of the following:

Neutral or slightly acid cake

Nongranular washing cream (no gumming or scrubbing)

If controlled peeling is employed, carefully verify the indications for sensitive skins before using

Conclude with a second warm atomization

Warm Vaporizer

Maximum of 10 minutes at a distance of about 15 to 20 inches from the face. It is also possible to apply warm compresses using a floral water (e.g., camomile infusions) .

Note. In the presence of redness or hypersensitivity, it is helpful to apply a cream before beginning while always taking care to remove the cream and to perform a third warm atomization after vaporization and before resuming treatment.

Extraction of Comedones and Milia

If necessary, proceed very delicately.

High Frequency

Use a violet ray electrode if the skin is flaccid.
If the skin is red or blotchy, use a neon ray electrode all around the red areas to create a decongestant effect by sparking.

Serum

If an oily serum is used, penetration can be enhanced by using manual massage (effleurage movements only). A serum is therefore selected with an azulene or similar base, which has a decongestant and softening effect.

If an aqueous serum is used, it will penetrate the skin by atomization or indirect massage (be cautious around reddened areas). A cream for sensitive skin will then be used for performing the massage.

Note. No pinching, slapping, cupping glass, or any other harsh treatment on blotchy skin.

Mask

A mask with bandelettes can be used if the skin lacks firmness or is beginning to show signs of flaccidity.

A moisturizing mask can also be used or a mask for diffuse redness or blotchiness.

Imbibition

Use a protective or night (treatment) cream with an azulene, hamamelis, or similar base.

Advice for the Client

Cleanse the skin well every morning and evening with a cleansing milk and appropriate lotion. Always avoid the use of soap or any lotion containing alcohol for cleansing the face. Avoid using water that is too hot or too cold, as well as saunas. Persons subject to redness in the skin must use decongestant creams and avoid overly long or harsh exposure to heat, cold, and wind. These persons must also eat lightly and avoid spicy foods and alcohol. Delicate or sensitive skins normally do not tan in the sun but burn easily; thus a good sun filter should be used with a horse chestnut or similar base. Persons with sensitive skin are well advised to stay in the sun only for very short periods of time.

TREATMENT FOR DRY OR ALIPOIDIC SKIN

Purpose of Treatment

To moisturize the skin

To activate secretions

To restore suppleness to the skin

Light Cleansing

Wash with:

Very light and unctuous cleansing milk with an almond or similar base

Lotion with a base of rose water

Initial warm atomization

Skin Analysis

The client's personal file

Deep Cleansing

Select from among the following:

Acidic or neutral cake
Nongranular washing cream (no scrubbing)
Controlled peeling (monitor the application time)
No galvanic disincrustation on this type of skin
Conclude treatment with a second warm atomization

Warm Vaporizer

From 12 to 15 minutes

Extraction of Comedones and Milia

If present

High Frequency

Spark with a violet ray electrode to obtain a bactericidal effect if comedones or milia have been extracted.

Activate circulation with an effluve from a neon ray electrode.

Serum

Apply a serum, preferably an oily type, and work it into the skin by manual massage.

If an aqueous serum is used, do a massage with a cream for sensitive skin. Remove the surplus before applying the mask.

Mask

Moisturizing mask of an algae or lecithin base

Imbibition

With a vitaminized cream made from a vegetable or animal oil base and containing vitamins A, E, and F

Advice for the Client

Thoroughly cleanse the skin in the morning and evening with a cleansing milk and a lotion appropriate for the particular skin type. If the skin is very dry, the use of a serum in the course of treatment is advisable. Take a treatment at the institute every week for about six weeks. Always use a protective moisturizing cream. Avoid using water with a high calcium content and alkaline products, soaps, and so forth. Always apply a sun filter (cream or oil) before exposing skin to the sun or a protective cream before exposure to cold and wind.

TREATMENT FOR COARSE, OILY SKIN

Purpose of Treatment

To curb secretions

To refine the skin

To constrict the ostia

To balance the pH

To brighten the complexion

Light Cleansing

Wash with:

Slightly acidic cleansing milk made from a grapefruit or currant base

Lotion with an orange or apple base

Initial warm atomization

Skin Analysis

The client's personal file

Deep Cleansing

Select from among the following:

- Galvanic disincrustation
- Granular washing cream (with scrubbing if skin is not sensitive)
- Controlled peeling
- Gumming mask
- Conclude with a second warm atomization

Warm Vaporizer

From 15 to 20 minutes

Extraction of Comedones

Vacuum apparatus (suction of sebum), large Jacquet pinchings, manual extraction

High Frequency

Spark with a violet ray electrode for a bactericidal effect following extraction.

Activate circulation with a neon ray electrode.

Serum

Apply a serum, preferably an aqueous one, made from a yeast, lemon, artichoke, or similar base to control secretions.

Mask

A mask for oily skin made with a fruit, lemon, or similar base or an artichoke base to brighten the complexion

Imbibition

With a protective nongreasy cream

Advice for the Client

Cleanse well in the morning and evening with a cleansing milk and a lotion appropriate for the skin type; never use irritating products such as soaps, or alcohol. If the skin is not sensitive, a granular or nongranular washing cream may be used two or three times per week. Always use a protective cream.

Once or twice a week, apply a serum followed by a mask to reduce secretions. If the skin shows a tendency to age prematurely, apply a treatment cream two to three times a week. It is advisable to take a treatment at the institute every 15 days or once a month. In serious cases (internal causes), advise the client to have a medical examination. The coarse, oily type of skin withstands the effects of the sun very well, nevertheless, the client should still be advised to use a sun milk or lotion.

TREATMENT FOR OILY SKIN WITH BLACKHEADS (COMEDONES)

Purpose of Treatment

To deep cleanse

To improve skin respiration

To refine the skin

To soften the comedones and dilate the ostia to facilitate extraction of the comedones (blackheads)

To normalize secretions

Light Cleansing

Wash with:

Cleansing milk made from a currant or similar base

A lotion with a thyme, camphor, or similar base

Initial warm atomization

Skin Analysis

Personal file of the client

Deep Cleansing

Select from among the following:

Galvanic disincrustation

Light peeling

Granular or nongranular washing creams (scrubbing if the skin is not too sensitive)

Gumming mask, warm paraffin mask, and so forth

Conclude with a second warm atomization

Warm Vaporizer

From 15 to 20 minutes. The esthetician can employ a manual massage using an oily cream to soften the comedones. Follow with a light cleansing milk or lotion to remove the oily residue that would interfere with the extraction of the comedones and subsequent treatments.

Extraction of Comedones

Vacuum apparatus (suction of sebum), large Jacquet pinchings, manual extraction. The extraction procedure should not last longer than 15 minutes.

High Frequency

Spark with a violet ray electrode to disinfect areas where comedones were removed.

Serum

Atomize with an aqueous serum made with a yeast or similar base or application and penetration by ionization of an ionizable serum appropriate for this type of skin.

Mask

Apply a mask with an artichoke or similar base, which will help brighten the complexion, or a moisturizing mask if the skin is dehydrated.

Imbibition

With a moisturizing cream

Note. With this type of skin, never use astringent products before having first completely freed the skin of comedones.

Advice for the Client

Perform a light cleansing every morning and evening with a cleansing milk and a lotion appropriate for this skin type. If the skin is not too sensitive, recommend a granular or nongranular washing cream as a replacement for the milk and lotion for cleansing at home, or alternate the two. Use a slightly acidic protective cream. One treatment per week at the institute is advisable until the skin is completely free of comedones. Never use astringent products before the end of the series of treatments at the institute or before the skin is totally clean. In serious cases (internal causes) , advise the client to have a medical examination. Greasy foods, chocolate, soft drinks, and so forth, should be avoided. If the client is exposed to the sun, advise her to use a sun filter (milk or lotion); avoid the oils.

TREATMENT FOR ASPHYXIC SKIN

Purpose of Treatment

To free the skin in order to permit normal respiration

To brighten the complexion

To refine the skin and normalize the texture

To remoisturize the skin if necessary

Light Cleansing

Wash with:

A mild cleansing milk because this type of skin is often dehydrated

Very mild, nonastringent lotion

Initial warm atomization

Skin Analysis

Personal file of the client

Deep Cleansing

Select from among the following:

Light peeling, gumming mask

Granular or nongranular washing creams (with scrubbing of the skin if not too sensitive)

Complete the treatment with a second warm atomization

Warm Vaporizer

From 15 to 20 minutes. The esthetician can proceed to a manual massage with an oily cream to soften the comedones. Follow with a light cleansing (milk or lotion) to remove the residue that would interfere with the extraction of comedones and the remainder of treatment.

Extraction of Comedones, Sebaceous Cysts, Milia

For a maximum duration of 15 minutes

Note. The esthetician must never extract sensitive, large, or deep cysts because they must be treated medically.

High Frequency

Spark with a violet ray electrode to disinfect regions where comedones were removed.

Serum

Atomize and penetrate by indirect massage of an aqueous serum made with a yeast or similar base. An appropriate ionizable serum for this type of skin can also be applied and worked into the skin by ionization.

Mask

An oxygenating mask or a moisturizing mask is preferable

Imbibition

With a vitaminized or moisturizing cream

Advice for the Client

Cleanse the skin every morning and evening with a cleansing milk followed by a lotion appropriate for this type of skin. If the skin is not too sensitive, the use of a granular washing cream is recommended two to four times a week. Weekly treatments in the institute are advisable until the skin is completely cleared. Never use astringent products. Always use a moisturizing protective cream until secretions normalize. After exposure to the sun, cleanse the skin well to remove the protective product used and apply a moisturizing cream.

TREATMENT FOR AGING SKIN

Purpose of Treatment

To detoxicate and deep cleanse the skin in order to eliminate dead cells and activate metabolism

To remoisturize the skin to eliminate lines and prevent new wrinkles from forming

To restore the skin's firmness

To combat sagging

To stimulate circulation

To restore the skin's radiance

Light Cleansing

Wash with:

A cleansing milk appropriate for this skin type

Toning lotion

Initial warm atomization

Skin Analysis

Personal file of the client

Deep Cleansing

Select from among the following:
Light peeling, washing cream. If the skin is coarse, a gumming mask can be used. If the skin is oily or greasy, the esthetician can proceed to a galvanic disincrustation if there are no pimples or acne rosacea condition. Complete the treatment with a second warm atomization.

Warm Vaporizer

From 15 to 20 minutes

Extraction of Comedones

If necessary

High Frequency

With a violet ray electrode to achieve a toning and bactericidal effect. Activate the circulation with a neon ray electrode. If there are bags below the eyes, the eyelid electrode can be used over a tissue.

Vacuum Apparatus

Work on all wrinkles very thoroughly using a cupping glass.

Serum

Apply an aqueous, oily, lyophilized or ionizable serum made from a collagen, connective tissue, embryonic, or similar base. Perform a manual massage with an oily serum or nourishing cream, using the firming manipulations. Conclude this massage with effleurage motions.

Mask

Apply a moisturizing mask or a mask that will counteract wrinkles. The use of bandelettes is often very effective.

Imbibition

Using a moisturizing cream

Advice for the Client

Cleanse the skin well in the morning and evening with a cleansing milk, followed by an appropriate lotion for this type of skin. Regular treatments at the institute are advisable, to be followed by appropriate measures at home. Once or twice a week, a serum should be applied, followed by a mask. Drink a lot of water, and avoid excessive alcohol and smoking. Sleep at least eight hours every night. Always apply a protective cream in the morning and a nourishing cream in the evening. If the skin is sagging, massage with a firming cream. The esthetician will demonstrate how to perform these massages. Before exposing skin to the sun, always apply a sun filter and be certain to remoisturize the skin after every exposure. If there are any major problems, advise the client to seek medical attention.

TREATMENT FOR ACNE-PRONE SKIN

Purpose of Treatment

To clean the deep tissues

To facilitate the free flow of sebum

To normalize secretions

To balance the skin's pH

To disinfect the skin

Light Cleansing

Wash with:

A cleansing milk from a camphor or similar base

Lotion made from a camphor base

Initial warm atomization

Skin Analysis

Personal file of the client

Deep Cleansing

Select from among the following:

Light peeling

Granular or nongranular washing cream, scrubbing
Acidic cake

Conclude with a second warm atomization.

Warm Vaporizer

From 15 to 20 minutes

Extraction of Comedones

Extract the comedones, which come easily; never force them unnecessarily, for this can harm the client's face by irritating the skin or leaving marks. Never touch nodules or pustules. If pus runs out during treatment, immediately clean the area with a little alcohol. The period used for extraction should never exceed 15 minutes. The vacuum apparatus may be used to facilitate extraction and remove excess sebum.

High Frequency

With a violet ray electrode, disinfect the regions where extractions took place by fulguration.

Serum

A serum made from a yeast base or any other serum that will help oxygenate the skin is recommended.

Note. Massage manipulations should be avoided with acne-prone skin.

Mask

Depending on the problem, apply a calming mask, or for redness, apply a mask with a hamamelis base; an artichoke base mask may be used for oxygenation or a fruit base mask for oily skin.

Note. Imbibition must not be performed with this type of skin.

Advice for the Client

Cleanse the face well every morning and evening with an acidic washing cream, or if the skin is too sensitive, alternate with a cleansing milk, followed by an appropriate lotion for this type of skin. Never scrape or press blackheads or pimples. Apply a protective cream every morning. It is advisable to have a treatment at the institute once every week until the skin is free of comedones, blackheads, and so forth. Throughout the period when the client is receiving treatment at the institute, she should apply the contents of one ampul of serum made from a yeast or similar base two or three times a week. If there are major problems, advise the client to seek medical attention.

14

Hair Removal (Depilation)

HAIR REMOVAL WITH HOT WAX

Hot wax to be used for the body, legs, thighs, arms, and so forth, is usually available in cakes or blocks weighing about two pounds (1 kg) ; wax for facial use is sold in small disks. The color of the wax varies according to which active ingredients are present (e.g., azulene, chlorophyll) .

Directions for Use

Melt the wax, let cool until lukewarm and keep it at the desired temperature.

Disinfect the area to be depilated with alcohol, and dry with a little talc to straighten the hair up again.

Before starting, the esthetician must test the temperature of the wax by placing a small amount on her wrist.

With a wooden spatula, turn the wax and spread a layer in the direction of hair growth while being careful to round out the edges so that it will hold well. (A strip should be 1½ to 2 inches wide.)

If the wax strip is too thin, thicken it with a second layer.

With the hands, press down on the wax so that it will adhere well.

Take hold of the rounded edge of the wax strip and pull it up with a rapid motion in the opposite direction from hair growth.

Rest the free hand firmly on the depilated area to reduce discomfort.

After the depilation has been completed, apply an azulene-base or similar soothing cream.

The same wax can be used several times for depilation of the body hair.

After the depilation, reheat the wax and filter it. Always use fresh wax for facial hair depilation.

Never boil the wax.

Note. Never remove hair where there are varicose veins, skin diseases, or injuries. Always use fresh wax for facial depilation.

HAIR REMOVAL WITH WARM WAX AND BANDELETTES

Warm wax is usually a vegetable wax and is packaged in different sized containers with bandelettes. The bandelettes come either in rolls about 2 inches wide or in strips 8 to 10 inches long and about 2 inches wide.

Directions for Use

Place the container of wax in boiling water, having first made sure to remove the lid.

Disinfect the portion to be depilated with alcohol and dry with a little talc (optional).

If the bandelettes are in rolls, cut several strips about 8 to 10 inches long.

When all the wax has melted reduce the heat, but keep the water warm so the wax will remain liquid for the duration of the procedure.

Dip a metal spatula into the liquid wax, and wipe off one side so only one side of the spatula has wax. Rapidly spread a thin layer of wax in the same direction as the hair grows while keeping the spatula at a right angle to the skin (not flat). In this way, coat the front of the leg along the length of a bandelette.

Without waiting, place a bandelette on the wax starting at the bottom of the leg.

Make the wax adhere well by smoothing it out firmly from bottom to top.

With one hand holding the skin, use the other to remove the bandelette with a single rapid movement in the opposite direction from hair growth. Rest the free hand firmly on the depilated area to reduce the discomfort. Immediately apply the same bandelette to the next area on another part of the wax coating; repeat the same procedure until all the wax that has been applied has been removed.

When the depilation has been completed, clean the depilated areas well with alcohol or a special solvent lotion to remove any wax residue.

Apply a soothing cream on the depilated areas.

Note. Never remove hair where there are varicose veins, skin diseases, or injuries.

15

Makeup

For each of us, makeup is a way of improving our appearance. Previously, it was used to cover defects, imperfections in the skin, and so forth, but sometimes with unfortunate results. Today, we begin by conditioning the skin before applying makeup. Makeup is more subtle, for we are always seeking the natural look that gives the skin a fresh, young appearance.

Makeup base and rouge play with effects of light and shadow: accentuate a hollow, shorten or refine the appearance of the nose, shade a particular feature, accent an expression or smile. The primary aim of makeup is to give the face character and to make it look pretty and alive.

In the following pages, several methods of applying makeup and of bringing about improvements will be discussed with a view of enhancing one's appearance under all kinds of conditions. We will also discuss color harmony and a few notions about the personalities attributed to different types and shapes of faces.

MORPHOLOGY

In makeup, morphology is the study of different facial shapes for the purpose of

1. Drawing psychological conclusions, such as determining a person's character;
2. Drawing esthetic conclusions to determine the weak points in a person's face and to initiate the appropriate corrections.

Faces can be divided into two main categories—angular and round.

Angular Faces

Angular faces are well delineated with a strong bone structure and musculature. Such faces lend themselves to light and shadow emphases. Within this category, there are the following facial forms and types:

Diamond-trapezoidal shape	Jupiter type
Rectangular shape	Saturn type
Rectangular shape	Mars type
Square shape	Earth type
Triangular shape	Mercury type

Round Faces

As the name suggests, this type of face has curved, continuous, and gently sloping lines without any bony projections. The following shapes and facial types are found in this category:

Oval shape	Apollo type
Round shape	Lunar type

Characteristics of several facial shapes and types are usually seen on any given individual. Very few people have a perfect facial shape.

Trapezoidal Shape (Jupiter Type)

The face is pear-shaped and wide with large sinewy features. The sides tend to thicken with age and become flabby. The inverse trapezoidal face has a more fully developed forehead than lower face; it is heavy with full but firm cheeks.

Personality. A Jupiter is an optimist. She loves to eat and drink and is comfortable with family and in society. She holds herself in high esteem and has no complexes; possesses a certain natural authority and can work very hard but in a very relaxed way. She loves luxury and honors; in other words, she has all the traits of a social climber; is much more sensual than sentimental.

Makeup. The steady aspect of this type of face can be maintained and harmonized. If the lower zone truly dominates the others, the upper zone should be emphasized and the lower zone deemphasized in order to give the appearance of an oval.

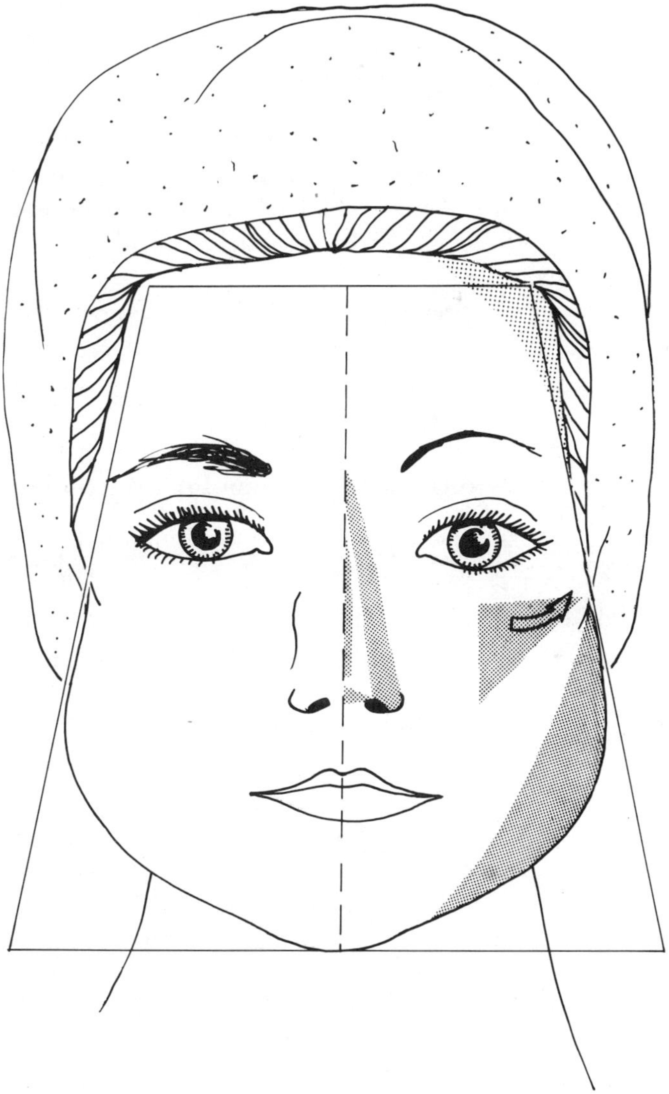

Rectangular (Saturn-Mars Type)

Elongated Rectangular (Saturn). The face is elongated in the shape of a rectangle and is lean and bony. It is very well delineated, longer than it is wide. The nose, forehead, and chin are all elongated and the mouth is thin.

Personality. Sense of humor is, like the complexion, more somber with an introverted character. Aggressive and stubborn; has few interests but always goes to the very core of a chosen subject. A specialist type.

Balanced Rectangular (Martian). This type of face is balanced with respect to length and width but the profile is angular. It is a face always well delineated, both from the front and the side.

Personality. Aggressive and stubborn, can also be violent, combative, impassioned, and impulsive. Has a solid intelligence but is subject to outbursts of passion.

Makeup. If the face is overly long, it must be made up to look broader and shorter. If the face is well balanced as to its length and width, it has harmony and there is no need to lengthen it. These types of faces must be brightened as much as possible, thus a luminous makeup base should be used.

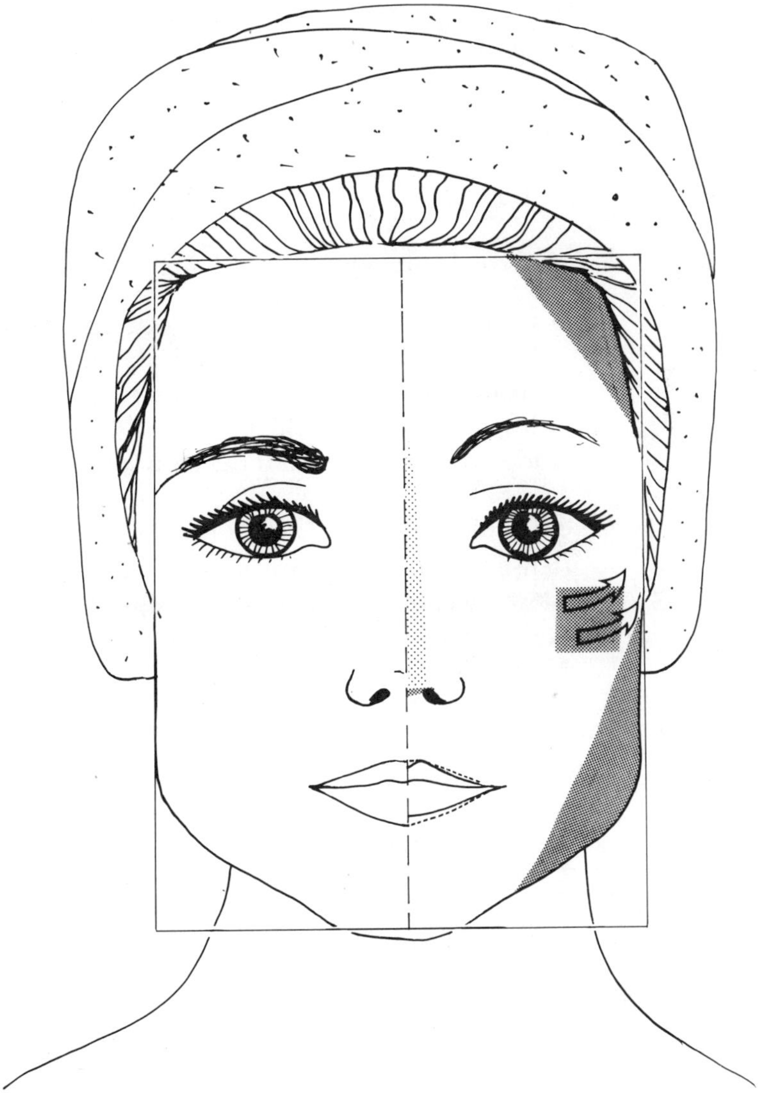

Square (Earth Type)

Face is cube-shaped with sharp angles and an unbalanced appearance. It is wider than it is long. Primitive type, short and thickset. The face is hard with a prominent high forehead. Eyes are recessed with small, straight thick eyebrows. The nose is flat (short, large, wide), the lips thick, and the chin square.

Personality. Instinctive behavior dominates. Has an intense desire to acquire material goods and pleasures. Follows a slow pace; has few ideas but completes what has been started. Has a strong will and perseveres. Possesses a great capacity for action; is a traditionalist.

Makeup. Primarily it is necessary to refine and soften the whole face—the mouth, nose, and so forth. One can also try to make the face up to look more oval. The makeup base must also be soft and light.

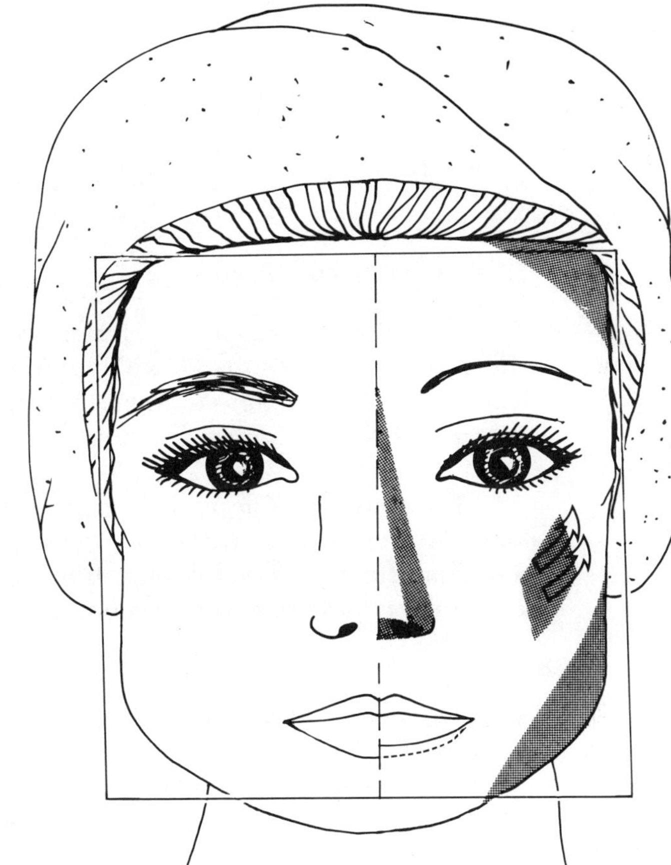

Triangular (Mercury Type)

The upper third of the face is more developed with respect to width and length, compared with the lower two-thirds of the face. The angles of the upper jaw, nose, and cheek bones are sharp. The nose and chin are pointed.

Personality. The type of person who is curious about all kinds of ideas and living things. Spontaneous, lively, gentle, unstable and unorganized; resourceful but unscrupulous; mentally and physically capable, very fast, but not very efficient.

Makeup. The face must be given more balance, by enlarging the base and deemphasizing the upper part of the face. The eyes and mouth should be enlarged, the chin and nose made shorter. A luminous makeup base should be used.

Oval (Apollo-Venus Type)

Apollo (Elongated Oval). Well-developed forehead, both in width and height, in keeping with the long lines of the face. Fine, classic features with a romantic expression.

Personality. Very sensitive, easily hurt; even tempered, slow to make friends, but very receptive to refined influences. Likes luxury, the arts, and people associated with the arts; artistic.

Venus (Short Oval, Heart Shaped). Hair forms a widow's peak. Eyebrows are very well arched; eyes are large and almond shaped. Heart-shaped sensual mouth. Expression is soft and languorous.

Personality. Gay and agreeable; very sensitive, sensual, emotional, and instinctive.

Makeup. To balance the elongated oval face, one can either shorten it at the chin and forehead or balance it by not lengthening it any further.

The short oval is already balanced in all three zones. This type of face can be accented, however, by emphasizing the mouth and eyes in their natural form. Character can be added to the face by refining the middle and lower zones to give the impression of a more triangular face.

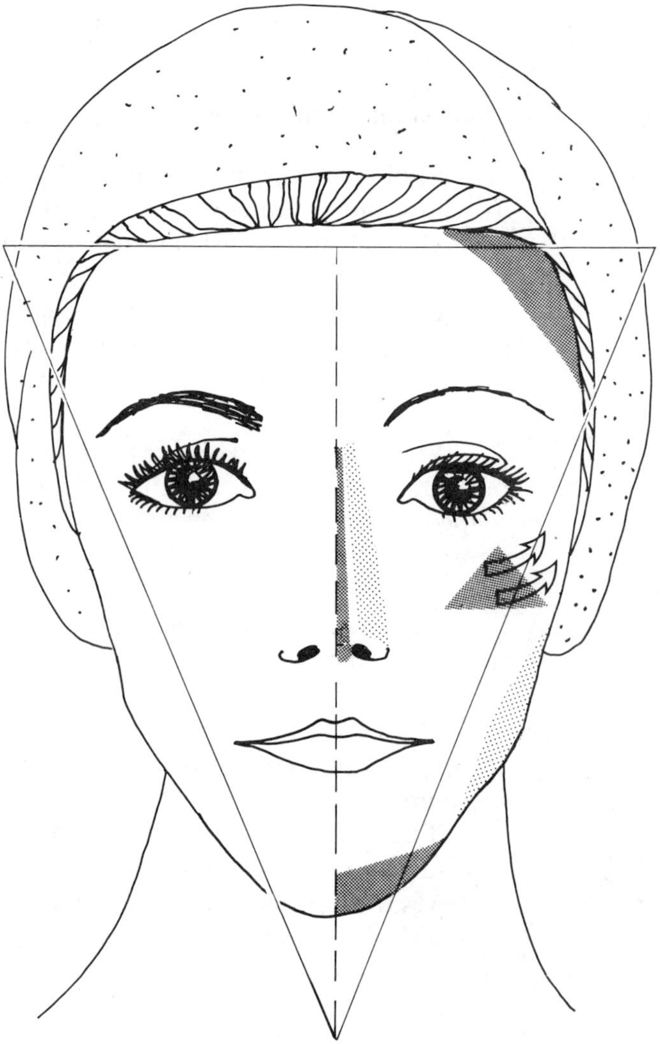

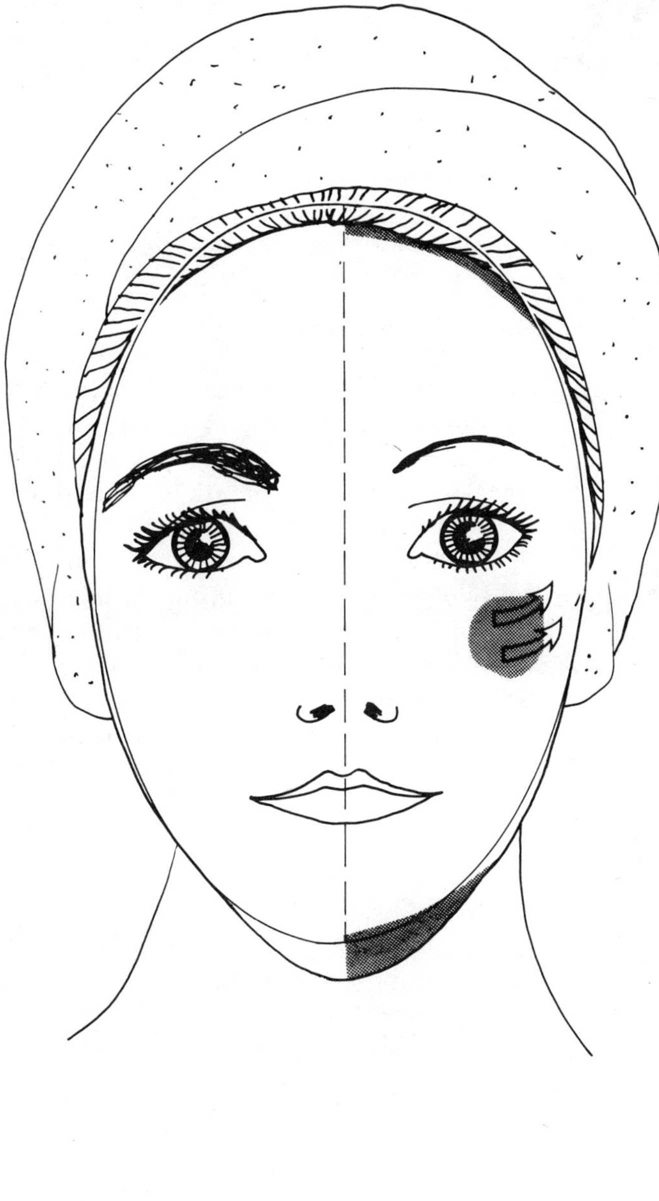

Round (Lunar Type)

This face has a babyish expression; it is round and remains round even with aging. The forehead dominates and the eyebrows are barely noticeable; the eyes are rounded, the nose flat, short, and turned up. The mouth is soft and pouty.

Personality. A true type would be indolent, lazy, thinking only of eating and drinking. Incapable of organizing his/her life. Fortunately, this type is only found in association with other types.

Makeup. The face should be balanced by elongating the lines slightly. The eyes and eyebrows should be darkened and a light bronze makeup base should be used.

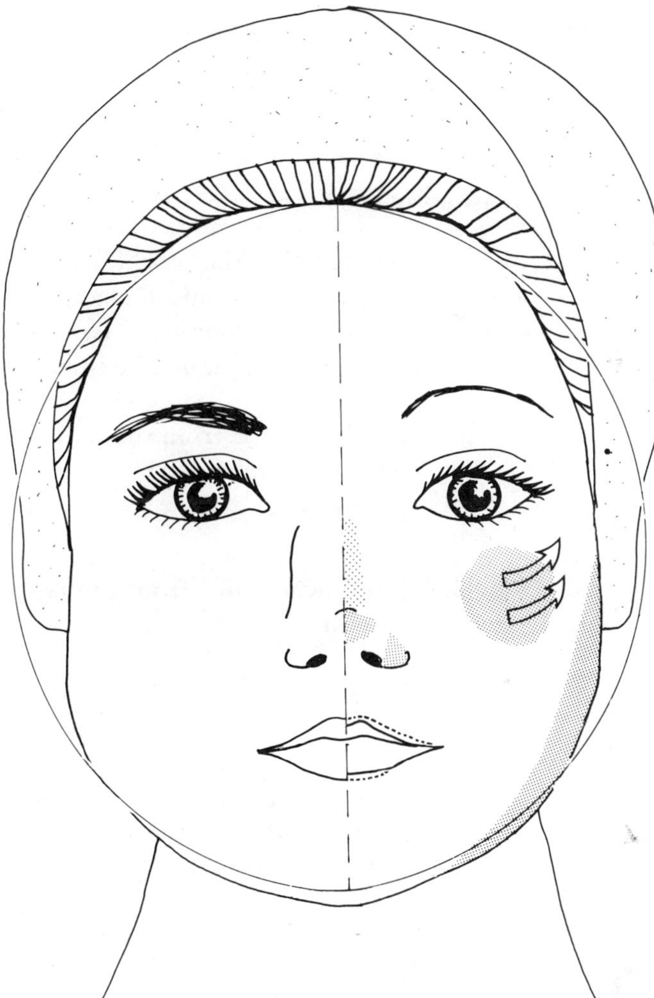

Divisions of the Face

In order to determine the morphological type of a particular face to be made up and the kinds of changes required, the face must be divided into three horizontal and two vertical zones.

On the horizontal plane, the three zones are

1. The forehead: from the hair to the base of the nose (between the eyebrows)
2. The middle zone: from the eyebrows to the end of the nose
3. The lower zone: from the end of the nose to the tip of the chin

There will be perfect facial harmony if the three zones are balanced.

On the vertical plane, a line is drawn down the center of the face from the hair to the chin. In this way, any asymmetry between the right and left side can be determined and corrected through the use of makeup.

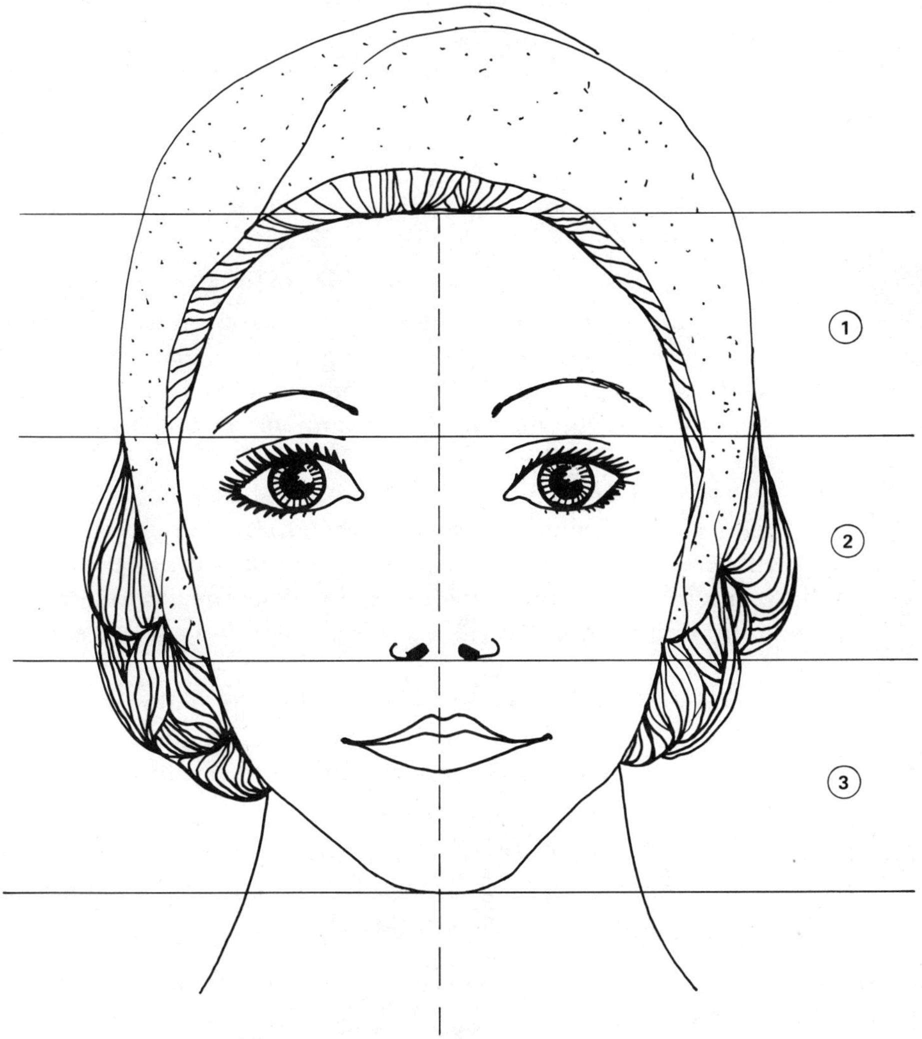
1
2
3

PLUCKING THE EYEBROWS

Before plucking the eyebrows, first decide what shape should be given to them and what corrections might be necessary in order for them to blend with the rest of the face.

The space between the eyebrows over the bridge of the nose can be determined by

1. The space between the eyes
2. The width of the nostrils

The average space between the eyebrows will be the same as the width of one eye. If the space is narrower than that, the eyebrows are too close together. If the existing space is equal to the width of the nostrils as well as the eye, the balance is perfect. If the width of the nostrils is uneven, the space between the eyes must serve as a guide.

The starting point of the eyebrow should be in line with the inside corner of the eye or with the outer crease of the nostril. If the two nostrils are not even, the starting point of the eyebrow is made from half way between the inside corner of the eye and the outer crease of the nostril. These steps should be followed:

1. Hold a pencil in the vertical position alongside the outer corner of the nostril; the point of the pencil will indicate the starting point of the arch of the eyebrow.
2. While making sure the eye is looking straight ahead, hold the pencil vertically and place it next to the outer curve of the iris. The tip of the pencil will indicate the uppermost point of the arc.

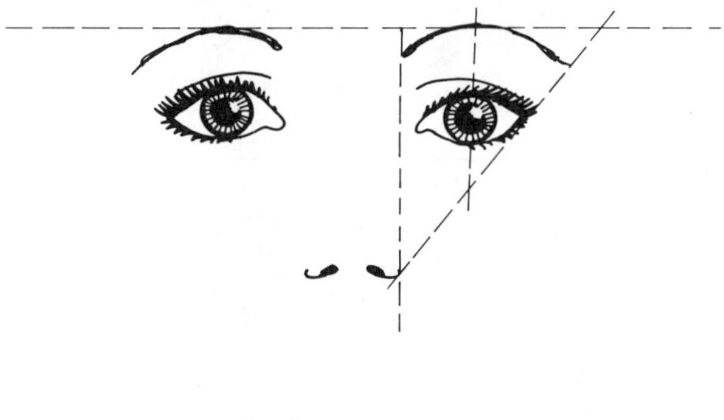

3. Slant the pencil from the outer corner of the nostril to the outer corner of the eye to show where the arch should end.
4. Test the height of the two eyebrow arches by placing the pencil horizontally over the eyebrows.

After the shape of the eyebrow has been determined and drawn, plucking may begin.

Necessary Accessories for Plucking the Eyebrows

1. Eyebrow brush
2. Eyebrow pencil
3. Tweezers

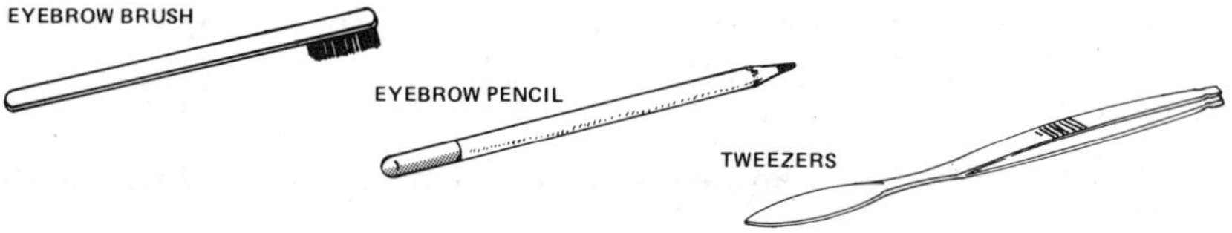

Care of the Accessories. Always disinfect the brush and tweezers after each plucking.

Note. Never apply a cream to the eyelid before plucking.

Procedure for Plucking

The area to be plucked should be well disinfected with alcohol. Brush the hairs with an eyebrow brush to smooth them. Stretch the skin firmly between the thumb and index finger, and begin plucking according to the desired shape. Pluck each hair individually with a quick, clean movement in the direction of hair growth. When completed, disinfect the area once again with alcohol and remove all pencil marks.

Finally, apply an azulene cream to soothe the skin.

Making Up the Eyebrows

After plucking, it is often necessary to improve upon the eyebrows by either filling them out or enlarging them to conform to the desired shape. Corrections are made using a sharpened pencil or a very fine brush and eyeliner. The color should match as closely as possible with the natural color of the eyebrows. Often, the best results are obtained when two colors are mixed together. The color should be applied in short, slanted strokes, each one representing a single hair. Finish by lightly brushing the brows in order to give them a more natural, soft look.

Appropriate Eyebrow Shapes for Each Facial Type

Trapezoidal—Jupiter. The eyebrow should not be too thick but slightly rounded and drawn out toward the temple.

Rectangular—Saturn, Mars. Eyebrows should be as natural as possible. Avoid a downward curve at the outer extremity and respect the space between the eyebrows over the bridge of the nose and the outer length.

Square—Earth. Fairly natural brow with a slightly rounded curve.

Triangular—Mercury. Brows should not be too thick or rounded. Often it is desirable to curve the brows upward slightly in order to emphasize the triangular shape of the face.

Oval—Apollo, Venus. The eyebrow should follow the natural line, that is, be parallel to the lid and drawn out toward the temple.

Round—Lunar. The eyebrow should be slightly arched; accent the curve somewhat in an oblique direction toward the temple.

COLOR HARMONY

In makeup, color harmony brings everything together, giving a well-coordinated, agreeable effect. The primary features whose colors must blend are the eyes, the hair, and the skin tone. It is important, too, that any makeup used enhance the person's natural coloration.

There are two basic color harmonies in makeup:

1. The bluish harmony—cold tones
2. The gold harmony—warm tones

In the bluish harmony (blue, mauve, pink, reddish-blue, gray) the following combinations are found:

Eyes	*Hair*
Blue or gray	Auburn, blue highlights (no yellow)
Black	Auburn, blue highlights (no yellow)
Blue or gray	Ash blonde
Blue or gray	Brown
Blue or gray	Silver

In the gold harmony (yellow, beige, orange, brown, green), the following combinations are found:

Eyes	*Hair*
Brown	Brown
Green	Brown
Green	Blonde
Green	Auburn, red highlights
Brown	Auburn, red highlights

For blue-green eyes (of changeable color), a color blend is selected according to the color of the hair and skin only.

The colors turquoise, aqua, white, and black belong to both color harmonies.

Factors which can change are:

1. Fashion and its color styles (these can be adapted to the person's age, profession, and facial shape)

2. Hair coloring
3. Tanning of the skin

Clothes and Color Harmony

It is very important to understand color harmony, for the color of one's clothes can show off one's personality to advantage. With a gold harmony, the colors such as yellow, orange, green, brown, and vermilion are best; with a bluish harmony, ones such as blue, gray, mauve, purple, bright pink, and wine red may be used.

People with white or gray hair should avoid using black near the face or any tan, brown, or gray colors. Any pastel color, however, suits them very well. Only people with black eyes and hair can wear any color from either of the two color harmonies.

APPLYING MAKEUP BASE

Since makeup is used to improve color, it is important to choose a makeup base that matches the skin tone. Makeup base comes in several consistencies: cake (compact) , cream, liquid. Generally, all contain the same basic ingredients, only the proportions vary. Liquid makeup bases are less concealing and thus look more natural. They are much creamier because they contain lanolin.

Before putting on any makeup, it is essential that the skin be clean. A protective cream should be applied first to prevent the makeup from being absorbed into the skin.

There are two types of make-up base:

1. A correcting base to improve poor skin tones
2. A harmony base that matches the natural skin tone

Selecting a Correcting Makeup Base

Green makeup base: to conceal red blotches, pimples, acne, and so forth

Mauve makeup base: to conceal poor skin tones, dullness, and paleness and to brighten the skin

Selecting a Harmony Make-up Base

A harmony makeup base must match the natural skin tone of the person as much as possible.

Bluish harmony: pinkish-beige, peach, or pinkish-ochre

Gold harmony: beige, brownish-gold, or ochre

Procedure

Makeup is smoothed on the face, always following the direction of the musculature as is done in facial cleansing. Makeup is applied in the following order: first, the correcting base, then an

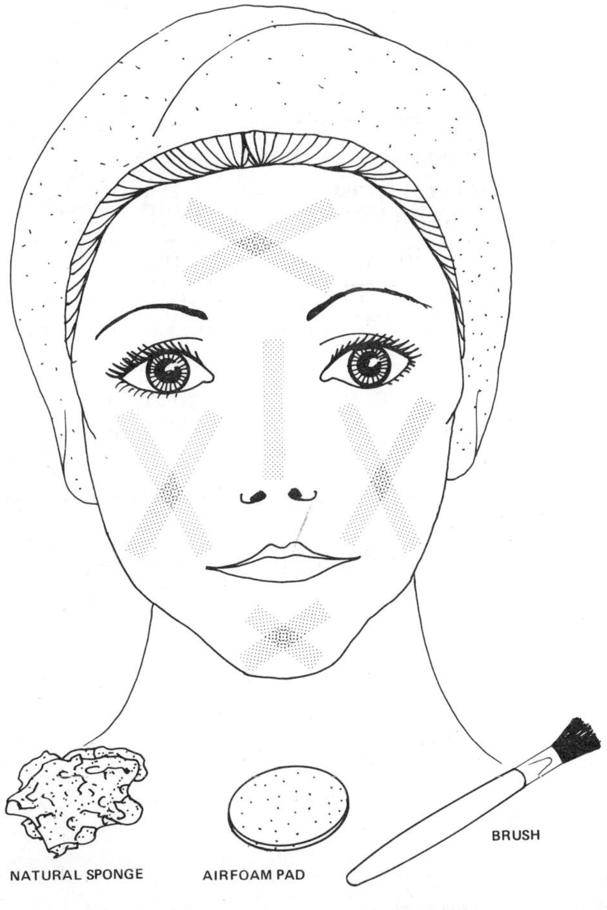

erasing cream to cover dark circles under the eyes, if necessary, and finally a harmony makeup base.

Correcting Makeup

Apply correcting makeup in small dabs using a thick makeup brush on the forehead, cheeks, nose, and chin. Then, with a damp sponge (from which any excess water has been removed by blotting it with a tissue) work in the color using light rapid strokes. Spread the color well over the entire surface of the face so that there are no lines at the neck, near the ears, or at the hairline.

Erasing Cream

After the correcting base, use an erasing cream to cover dark circles under the eyes. There are green-toned erasing creams as well as ones that are lighter in color than the makeup base. Both are available in various consistencies.

Harmony Makeup

Apply the harmony makeup base in the same manner as the correcting base. Finally, using an eyebrow brush, brush the brows in the opposite direction from the way they grow to remove any makeup that may have remained on them. Then smooth the brows back into their normal arch.

APPLYING ROUGE

Rouge also comes in the two color harmonies:

Bluish harmony: pink, reddish-blue, rose-beige

Gold harmony: coral, orange, reddish-brown

Rouge is applied to the cheeks with the fingertips in small amounts in the desired shape. If there is a surplus, remove very gently with a foam pad.

Application of Rouge for Different Facial Shapes

Facial Shape	Rouge Application
Trapezoidal	In a triangular shape with the wider part on top; shade toward the top 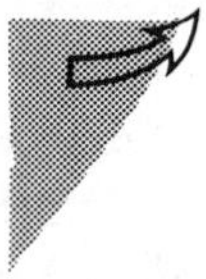
Elongated rectangular	In a horizontal rectangular shape in the center of the face; shade toward the outside and slightly upward 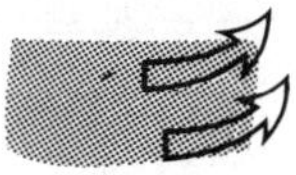
Balanced rectangular	Between the hollow and the bone structure
Square	In a slanted triangular shape; shade toward the top 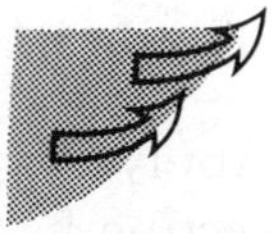
Triangular	In a triangular form, the large part on the bottom 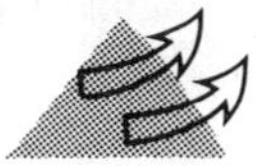
Oval	On the middle of the cheek 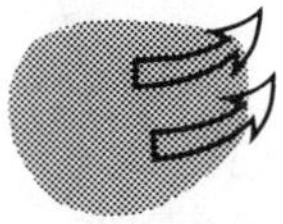
Round	In an elongated oval shape; shade toward the top 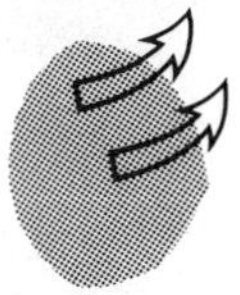

CORRECTIONS AND IMPROVEMENTS THROUGH THE USE OF MAKEUP

Corrections or improvements can be made using foundation, color makeup, special powder makeup, and a pencil. Dark makeup (bister or brown) reduces, and pale makeup (white or clear) enlarges. The latter also brightens, lengthens, fills out, and covers circles under the eyes and other imperfections. Bister or brown makeup reduces, deepens, darkens and conceals and is suitable for bags, hollow cheeks, and prominent cheekbones, large noses, chubby faces, and so forth.

When a cream makeup, a pencil, and a foundation are used, they must be used before powder is applied. If a powder makeup is used, it should be applied after powdering the face.

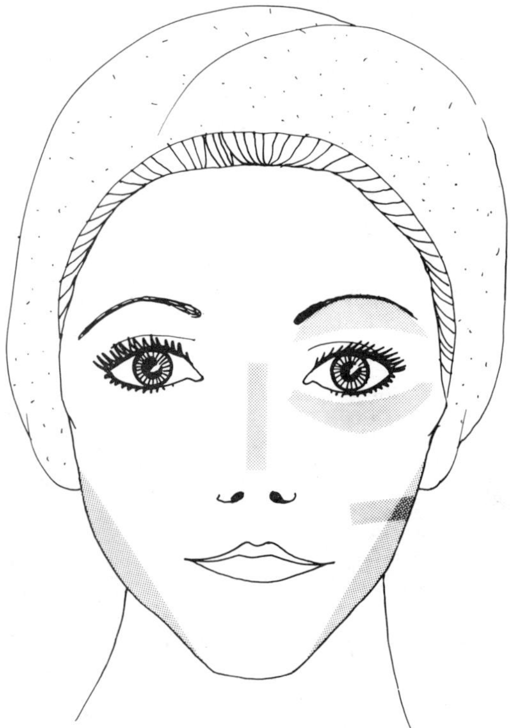

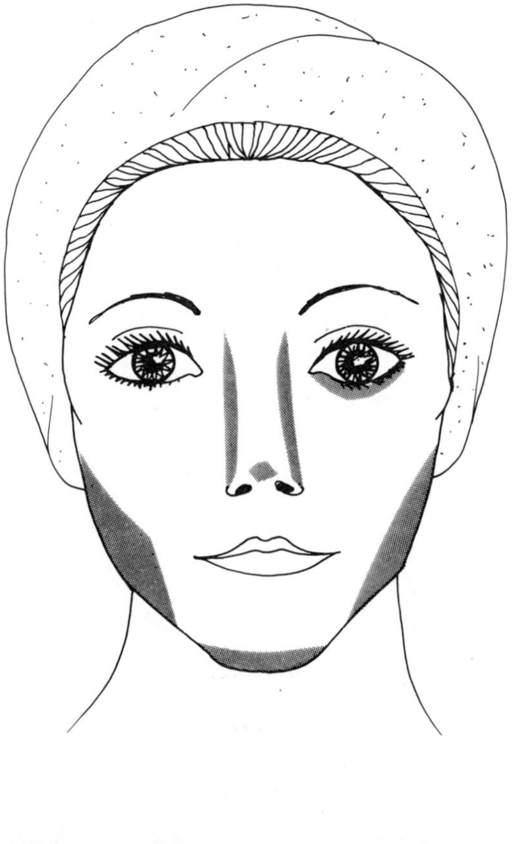

Correcting the Facial Form

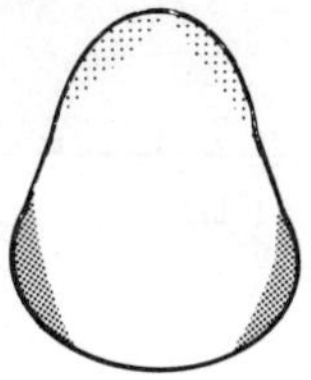

Trapezoidal—Jupiter. The lower part of the face is refined with a foundation or a bister makeup; the face can then be made to look more oval by using a white makeup at the temples.

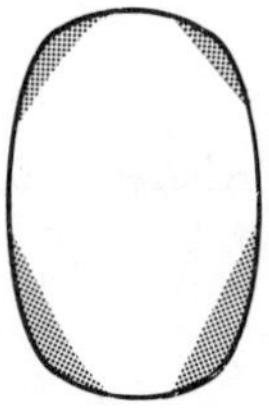

Rectangular—Saturn. The upper and lower face are refined with a foundation or bister makeup.

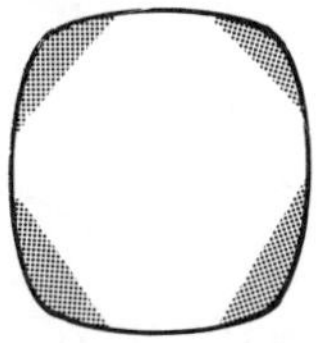

Square—Earth. Make the face look more oval by applying a foundation or bister makeup on the upper and lower parts of the face.

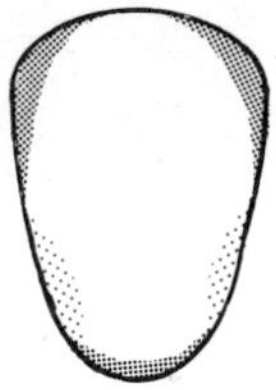

Triangular—Mercury. Refine the forehead using a foundation or bister makeup, and then enlarge the lower face using a white or pale makeup; finally, shorten the chin with a bister makeup.

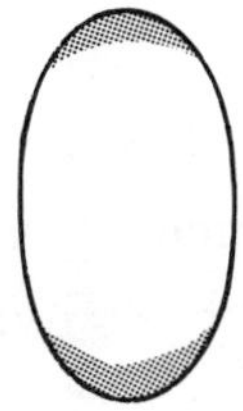

Long Oval—Apollo. Shorten the forehead and chin with a bister makeup or foundation.

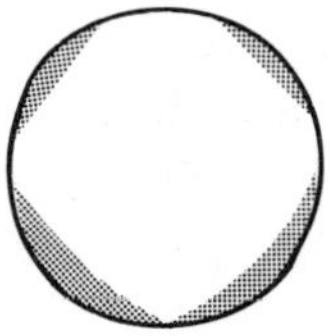

Round—Lunar. This facial form can be made more oval by using a bister makeup or foundation at the temples and around the lower part of the face.

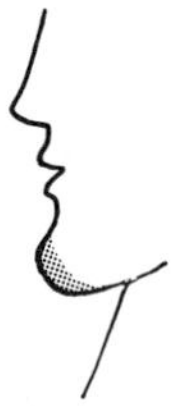

Correcting the Chin

Prominent Chin. A prominent chin can be corrected by applying a darker foundation or a bister makeup on the tip of the chin.

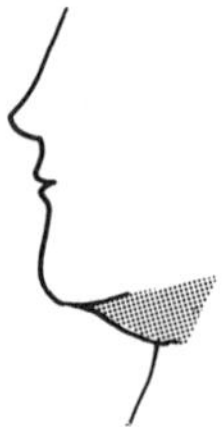

Double Chin. A double chin can be corrected by putting a bister makeup or foundation on the double chin.

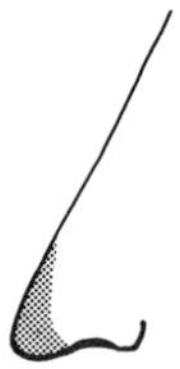

Correcting the Nose

Long Nose. Apply a foundation or bister makeup on the portion to be shortened.

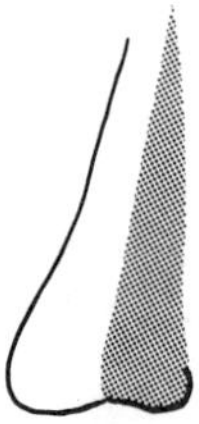

Broad Nose. Apply a foundation or bister makeup along each side of the nose.

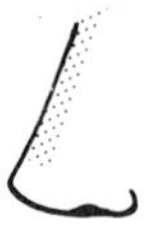

Short Nose. To give emphasis to a nose which is too small or too short, apply a bright foundation or a white or clear makeup along the top of the nose for its entire length.

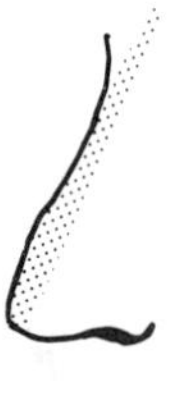

Crooked Nose. Draw a straight line in the middle and apply a bright foundation along this line; a darker foundation may be applied on the edge and on each side of the nose.

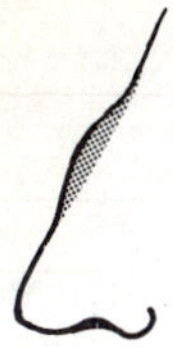

Nose with a Bump in the Middle. Apply a dark foundation or a bister makeup in a straight line on the bump.

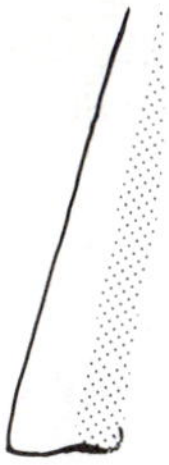

Narrow Nose. Apply a bright foundation or a white or clear makeup on each side of the nose.

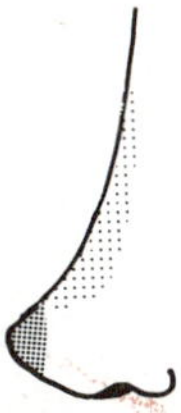

Turned-up (Pug) Nose. Apply a bright foundation or a white or clear makeup in the middle of the nose and a darker foundation or a bister makeup on the tip.

APPLYING POWDER

The purpose of powder is to set the foundation and makeup that have just been applied. A light translucent powder should be used. Dip a powder puff into the powder, shake off the excess, and without rubbing, pat it onto the face to firm or set the foundation and makeup. Remove any excess with a powder brush.

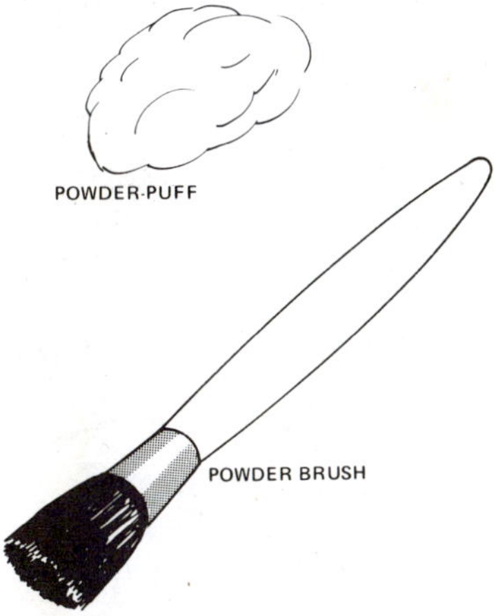

One can really use one's imagination with eye makeup. Nevertheless, before doing anything, it is necessary to decide how the eyes may be enhanced—by improving their shape if necessary, and, through the use of color, giving them a special brightness and beauty.

Almond-shaped eyes are considered to be the ideal shape. When making up the eyes, one tries, with the help of light and dark eyeshadow, eyeliner, pencils, and so forth, to make the necessary changes for each type of eye.

Different Shapes of Eyes and the Appropriate Corrections that Can Be Made with Makeup

Making Up Round or Protruding Eyes

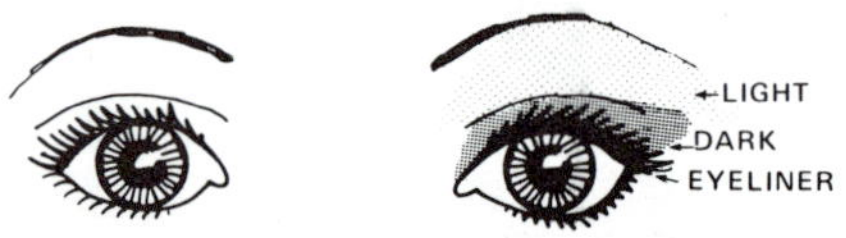

Making Up Deepset Eyes

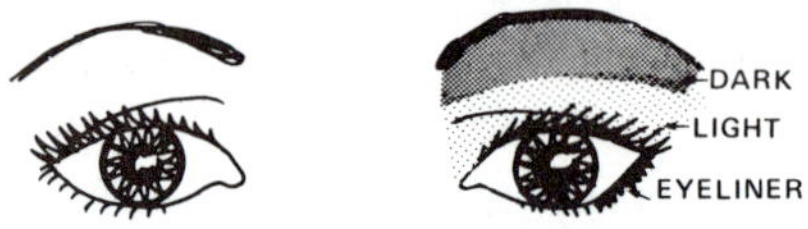

Making Up Drooping Eyes

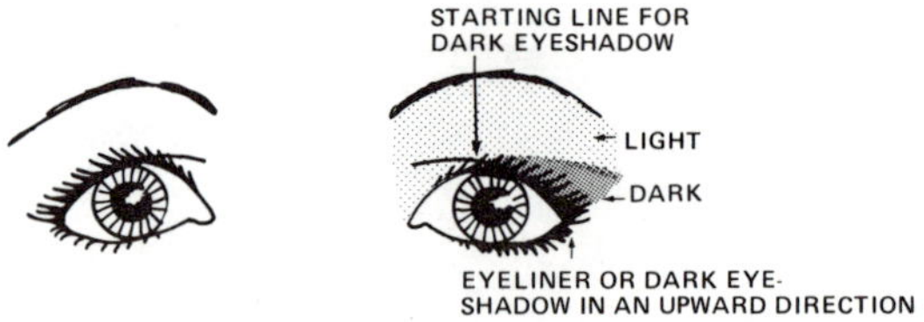

Making Up Almond-Shaped Eyes

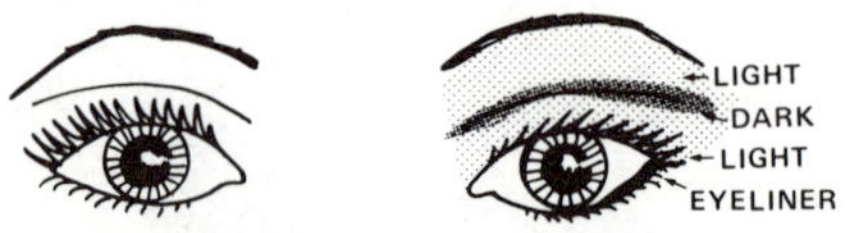

LIP MAKEUP

Determining the Correct Form

To determine the shape to be given to the lips or the corrections to be made, follow these three steps:

1. Place a pencil, with the point down, vertically over the center of the pupil of the eye. The tip of the pencil should be in line with the outside point of the lip and it should indicate the proper length to give to the mouth.
2. The projecting points of the upper lip should be in line with the center of each nostril.
3. The midpoint of the lower lip should be in line with the tip of the nose.

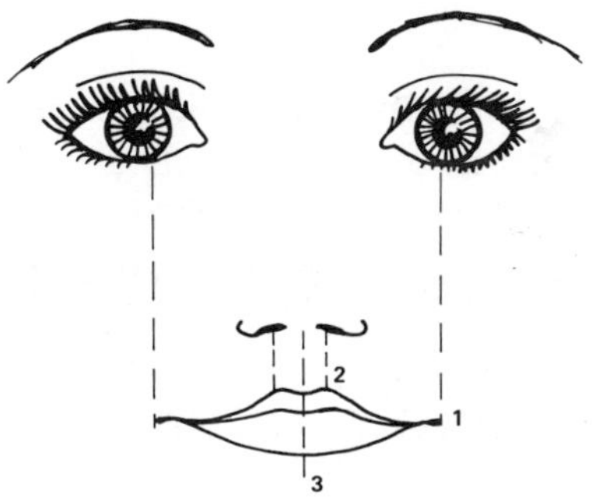

Procedure for Making Up the Lips

The lips should be well powdered before being made up. If the shape of the lips is to be corrected, it is preferable to first apply a foundation.

Using a pencil, outline the desired shape. Then, with a lip brush, apply a natural color (same as the color of the lips). Blot well with a tissue to remove any excess. Powder again and apply a lipstick selected according to the color harmony of the makeup.

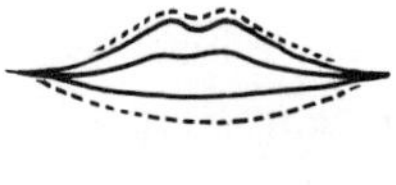

Thin Lips. Enlarge. Trace the desired shape with a pencil, apply the correcting color, blot, powder, and apply the appropriate harmony color.

Small Lips. Trace the desired shape with a pencil, apply the basic color, powder, and apply the appropriate harmony color.

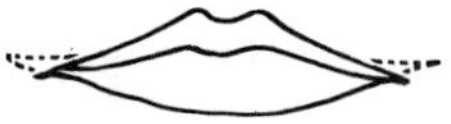

Downturned Lips. With a pencil, draw a more upturned shape, apply the correcting color, blot, powder, and apply the appropriate harmony color.

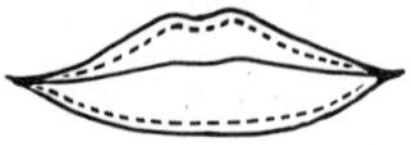

Thick Lips. Apply a makeup foundation to conceal the lip, powder, draw a line inside the natural lip line, and apply color keeping within the new line.

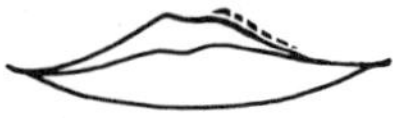

Asymmetric Lips. Apply a foundation; using a pencil, draw the necessary corrections, apply a basic color, blot, powder, and apply the appropriate harmony color.

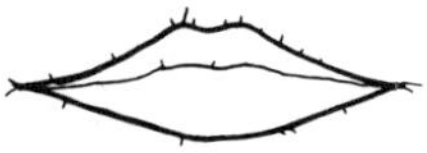

Wrinkled Lips. To correct wrinkles around the lips, proceed as follows: Apply a foundation on the lips and powder well. Outline the lips and put on lipstick, keeping it well within the line. Never use a lip brightener or lip gloss.

SETTING OR FIRMING MAKEUP

Once makeup has been applied, any excess powder must be removed to brighten its appearance. To do this, dampen a natural sponge (the same one used to apply the foundation) with very cold water, blot it with a tissue, and press it carefully over the entire face (NEVER RUB). This has the effect of setting or firming the makeup while removing any surplus powder.

If makeup has to be touched up during the day or evening, only powder makeup should be applied, using a makeup brush. Only one type of product should be applied with any one brush.

Caring for Makeup Brushes

Brushes Used for Liquid or Cream Makeup. Clean well using a cleansing milk until all of the color disappears, rinse in soapy water and then in fresh water; disinfect well. Always dry in the direction of the fibers.

Eyeliner Brushes. Wash in soapy water, rinse, and disinfect well. Dry in the direction of the fibers.

Dry Makeup Brushes, Eyebrow Brushes, Powder Brushes. Wash in soapy water, rinse, and dry well. Disinfect.

Puffs and Sponges. Wash in soapy water, rinse, and disinfect well.

APPLYING FALSE EYELASHES

False eyelashes are selected so that they match the color, shape, and expression of the eyes. They should also complement the individual's personality, age, and color harmony as well as the circumstances and places in which they are to be worn.

Fringed Eyelashes

1. Pick up the false eyelashes with the fingers and bend them around to make them more pliable and to give them the desired shape. The upper eyelashes are put on first.

2. Before putting on the glue, pick up the lashes with a tweezers and place them on the eyelid (no glue) to see if they have to be shortened to fit the length of the eyelid. If the false eyelashes are too long, the outer portion can be cut using a cuticle clipper.

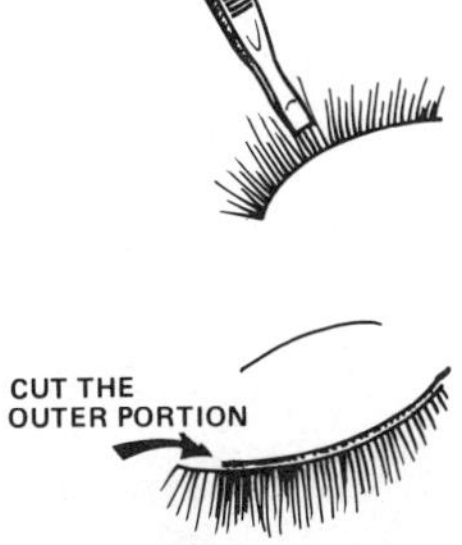

3. Place a small amount of false eyelash glue on the top of the hand. Using a small stick, spread a thin, uniform layer of glue over the entire length of the eyelashes.

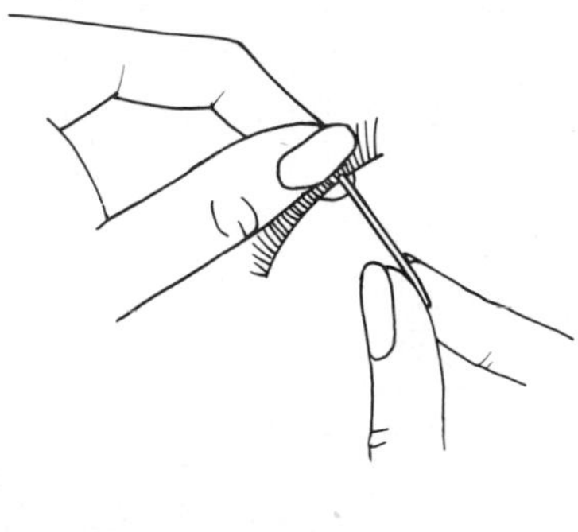

4. Next, take the eyelashes with a tweezers and place them on the eyelid at the very base of the natural lashes, leaving ¼ inch at the inside corner of the natural lashes. With the stick or the handle end of the tweezers, arrange the eyelashes in place before the glue dries.

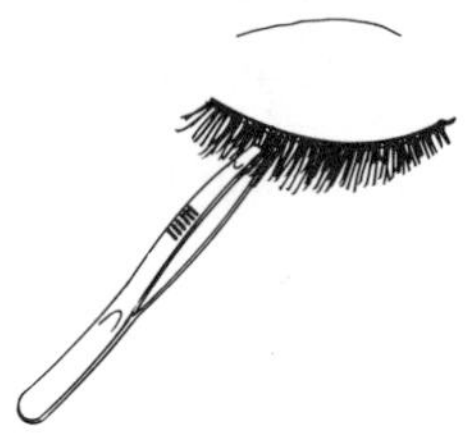

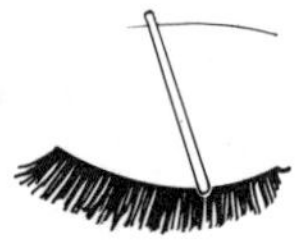

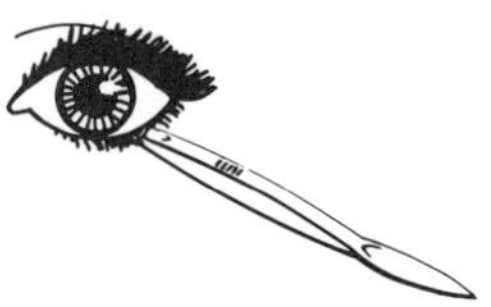

5. The lower eyelash can now be put on following the same procedure. Once the lower lash has been placed on the eyelid and before the glue dries, push the eyelashes carefully into place with the tweezers so that they are as close as possible to the base of the natural lashes. This also gives them a rounded shape.
6. A small amount of eyeliner can be added to fill in the inside corner of the eye, starting at the point where the lower lashes end up to the place where the upper lashes begin.
7. To remove false eyelashes, draw the eyelid out toward the temple and, using the tweezers, pull off the lashes starting at the outer corner and moving toward the inside.

Individual False Eyelashes (Single Lashes)

Using a cuticle clipper, separate the false lashes into small tufts of two to three lashes and place them on a tissue. If they are the same length, they should be cut to different lengths to give them as natural an appearance as possible. They must be longer near the outer portion of the eye and shorter towards the inside. Place some glue on your hand, and using a pair of tweezers, pick up the lashes and dip the base of the lashes in the glue until they are well soaked. Place the false eyelashes at the base of the natural eyelashes. Pick up another tuft and continue in the same way for the rest of the upper and lower lids. Single false eyelashes can be kept in place several days as long as the eyes are cleansed with a special lotion and not with ordinary oil.

EYELASH DYEING

To dye eyelashes, proceed as follows:

1. Cleanse carefully around the eyes.
2. With a makeup brush, apply a bit of petroleum jelly on the upper and lower eyelids. Be careful not to get any on the eyelashes.

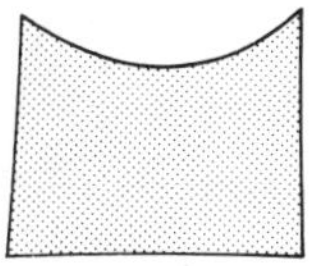

3. Cut two round pieces out of tissue paper, in the shape of an eye.
4. Place one piece under the lower lid. It will stick to the jelly.
5. Prepare the dye according to the manufacturer's directions.
6. Open the eye, and with a small flat brush or a small applicator stick, apply the dye on the lower lashes being careful not to touch the skin.
7. Then close the eye and apply the product on the upper lashes.
8. The manufacturer's directions will indicate how much to apply and how long to leave it.
   NOTE: IF A BURNING SENSATION IS FELT, REMOVE THE PRODUCT IMMEDIATELY AND WASH THE EYES WITH COLD WATER.
9. When finished, remove any excess with a dry cotton swab and then with a moist piece of cotton.
10. Clean the eyelids, taking care to remove all the jelly.
11. Wash the eyes with cold water.

MAKEUP FOR MEN

Although makeup for men follows the same principles as women's makeup, it is much more discreet.

1. If the eyebrows are to be plucked, they should not be made too thin, and their original shape should be maintained. Only individual hairs that are too long or those growing over the bridge of the nose should be removed. Take care to brush the brows well and, if necessary, to smooth them after completing the makeup.
2. Apply a protective cream.
3. If necessary, apply a correcting foundation and an erasing cream to conceal circles under the eyes.
4. The harmony foundation should be translucent and match the natural skin tone as closely as possible. Avoid using a pink-toned foundation.
5. Rouge must be very light, and only brown tones should be used.
6. If the face needs to be made to look more oval or refined or if the nose or chin need to be enlarged or shortened, proceed in the same way as outlined in the section Corrections and Improvements.
7. Powder the makeup with a translucent powder, making sure that any excess is removed. Brush the eyebrows, lashes, and moustache, if there is one, to remove any remaining particles of powder.
8. The eyes can be lightly outlined with an eyeliner or a pencil. If eyeshadow is used, keep to brown and gray tones; other shades are to be avoided.
9. The eyelashes and eyebrows can be made up with a special noncolored mascara or a mascara of the same color as the lashes and brows. They can be smoothed with a bit of soap and water.
10. The lips must be well cleansed with no traces left of powder or foundation. If desired, apply neutral colored or pale brown lipstick. A creamy lip gloss can also be applied.

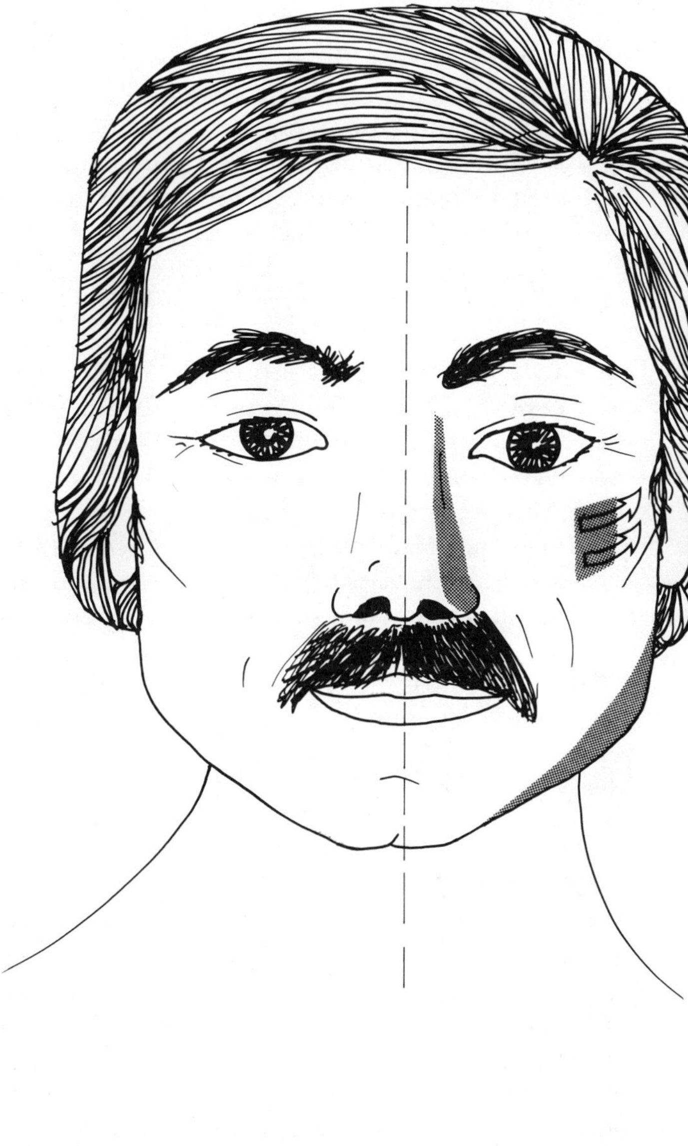

Note: The eyebrows, eyelashes, and moustache can be dyed in the same way as outlined in the section Eyelash Dyeing.

PRACTICAL TIPS

If you are about to make up a young girl who has never before been made up, BE CAREFUL. Be very gentle when plucking the eyebrows. Use a foundation if necessary. Rouge and lipstick may be applied with just a touch of eyeshadow and mascara. For a young woman in her twenties, accent her type of face, but here again, BE CAREFUL if she has never before used makeup. Do not use too elaborate a makeup, but proceed in gradual stages. A woman in her thirties can use a more sophisticated type of makeup as long as she is accustomed to using cosmetics. Again, BE CAREFUL, a client will frequently request a certain type of makeup currently in fashion that will not suit her. Know how to advise her.

After the age of 50, makeup must be light and soft, according to the fashion. If the client's hair is light, select clear colors, for a makeup which is too dark will harden her features. With persons over 65 years of age, caution must be exercised with faces that are too wrinkled. In such cases, it is often better to advise against the use of a foundation. A cream should be applied first, followed by a light powder, the same color as the complexion, a little rouge, and a light lipstick. This will make the face look brighter. Avoid making up the eyes. Pluck the eyebrows and fill them in lightly using natural tones. A light touch of mascara can be used. Makeup for older women is more discreet.

ANALYZING THE FACE BEFORE APPLYING MAKEUP

Survey the body and face as a whole. Note the proportions of the face and neck, the color of the skin (complexion), and the shape of the face (angular or rounded). Check to see if the three horizontal portions of the face are balanced (the forehead with the other two portions). Also check the vertical balance (width).

Compare the nose to the face as a whole. Is it in proportion, too small, too long, too wide? What corrections are necessary? Check the thickness, shape, and length of the mouth. Is the chin too pointed, double? Check the color and shape of the eyes. Are they small, rounded, down turned?

Finally, look at the color of the person's clothing. This must be taken into consideration when selecting colors of makeup.

THE ORDER OF APPLYING MAKEUP

Makeup should be applied in the following sequence:

1. Plucking eyebrows if necessary
2. Protective cream
3. Corrective foundation, concealing shadows under the eyes if necessary
4. Harmony foundation
5. Color makeup (rouge, and so forth)
6. Improvements, corrections
7. Powder
8. Eye makeup
9. Lipstick
10. Setting or firming makeup
11. Applying false eyelashes if desired

Whenever touch-ups are necessary, only dry makeup should be used.

Glossary

Abnormalities: Irregularities, imperfections.

Acidic: Having the properties of an acid, sour-tasting substance. Example: lemon juice.

Acne, Acneic: A common skin disease, especially among adolescents and young adults, characterized by chronic inflammation of the sebaceous glands, usually causing pimples on the face, back, and chest.

Albinism: The condition of being an albino. A person whose skin, hair, and eyes lack normal coloration because of genetic factors. Albinos have a white skin, whitish hair, and pink eyes.

Albumin: An organic substance, containing nitrogen, which is found in milk, egg, muscle, blood, and in many vegetable tissues and fluids.

Alipoidic: Lacking fat. Synonym: hypolipoidic.

Alkali: Any base or hydroxide that is soluble in water and gives a high concentration of hydroxyl ions in solution.

Alkaline: The opposite of acidic. Bitter-tasting substance, having the properties of an alkali. Examples: soda, potassium hydroxide, ammonia.

Allergy: A hypersensitive reaction to certain substances, foods, or products.

Alternating (Current): An electric current that reverses direction periodically.

Amidon (Starch): Organic substance (glucide) found in many vegetable foods, such as potatoes, wheat, corn. It is a granular solid.

Amino Acids: A group of nitrogenous organic compounds that serve as the unit structure of the proteins and are essential to human metabolism.

Angioma: A tumor made up mainly of blood vessels and lymph vessels.

Anion: A negatively charged ion.

Antibodies: Protein produced in the body to fight allergies, diseases, and germs.

Anti-Inflammatory: A substance that counteracts inflammation, reduces swelling and redness, and so forth.

Antiseptic: A substance that inhibits the growth or effects of bacteria.

Aqueous: Of, like, or containing water; water-soluble substance.

Argile (Clay): A firm, unctuous, fine-grained earth, composed mainly of aluminum silicates; easily malleable when wet.

Arterioles: Any of the smaller blood vessels, intermediate in size and position between arteries and capillaries.

Asphyxial: That which is blocked or unable to breathe.

Aster: A star-shaped structure, formed around the centrosome in the cytoplasm of any human or animal cell during mitosis.

Astringent: A substance that contracts body tissues and inhibits glandular secretions.

Atom: Any of the smallest particles of an element that combine with similar particles of other elements to produce compounds.

Atomize: To reduce a liquid to a fine spray.

Azulene: Active extract taken from the camomile (chamomile) plant or flower. Has a soothing effect.

Bactericidal: Containing an agent or substance that destroys bacteria. Example: alcohol.

Bandelettes: Strips of cotton cut to desired width and length.

Beaker: A small glass or metal container with a lip for pouring.

Biology: The science that deals with the origin, history, physical characteristics, life processes, habits, and so forth, of plants and animals.

Blotchy: Permanent dilation of the capillaries.

Calming: Sedative; reduces and relieves pain.

Camphor: A volatile, crystalline substance, derived from the camphor tree. Has a strong, characteristic odor. Used as an antiseptic.

Capillaries: Any of the tiny blood vessels connecting the arteries with the veins.

Cation: A positively charged ion.

Cellulitis: Inflammation of connective tissue, especially of subcutaneous tissue caused by infiltration of water, liquids, fatty substances, and waste at the level of the hypodermis.

Chloasma: Pigmentary patch, brownish in color, irregular in shape and size. Usually appearing on the face.

Chlorophyll: The green pigment found in plant cells.

Cholesterol: A crystalline fatty alcohol usually found in animal fats, blood, nerve tissue, and in higher levels, in bile.

Cicatrizant (Cicatrizing): That which has a healing effect, followed by the formation of a scar.

Claustrophobia: Feeling of anxiety; abnormal fear of being in an enclosed or confined place.

Collagen: A fibrous protein found in connective tissue.

Colloidal: Substance having the appearance of gelatin, gum, and so forth.

Comedo: A plug of dirt and fatty material that blocks the canal of the pilosebaceous gland. Often oxidizes to form a blackhead.

Convergent Lens: A piece of glass that brings together parallel rays of light, which, passing through it, are directed toward a common point.

Cosmetics: Substance or preparation designed to beautify, purify, or cleanse the skin, hair, and so forth.

Dartre (Tetter): Desquamation, flakes, scales, caused by certain skin diseases.

Décolleté: Area comprising the top part of the back, shoulders, neck, and chest.

Degenerate: Alteration, aging of the living cell.

Depurative: Purifying. A substance that helps clear all toxic substances and impurities from the blood.

Desquamative Layer: The most exterior layer of the skin, which peels or scales off.

Detergent: A cleansing substance.

Diffusion: Distribution of a substance in the body.

Diuretic: A substance that acts upon the urinary system, increasing the secretion and flow of urine.

Drain: To empty, or to draw water from, for cleaning.

Dual Emulsion: An emulsion containing two basic elements of a different nature.

Dyschromia: Abnormal pigmentation of the skin.

Effleurage: Light smooth massage; touching lightly.

Electrode: Any terminal tube or part that conducts an electric current into or away from an apparatus that is used to apply a treatment to the body.

Electron: An elementary particle of all atoms. It carries a negative electrical charge.

Embryonic Extracts: Extracts of any living thing in its earliest, most rudimentary stage of life. Example: chicken embryo.

Emollient: Any softening or soothing substance that has a tissular relaxing effect and relieves inflammation.

Energy: Potential forces; inherent powers.

Enzymes: Any of various proteinlike substances found in plant and animal cells that act as organic catalysts in initiating or speeding up specific chemical reactions.

Ephelides (Freckles): Small brownish spots on the skin, usually appearing as a result of exposure to the sun.

Essential Oils (Volatile oils—Essence): Oils obtained through the distillation of aromatic substances extracted from various plants.

Esthetician (Aesthetician): Student or expert in the field of esthetics. Person whose profession consists of giving skin care treatments for the purpose of normalizing nonpathological alterations of the skin.

Evanescent: Tending to fade away, gradually disappearing or vanishing.

Flabbiness: Lack of firmness; atonicity.

Flaccidity: Softness; looseness; lack of force, firmness.

Galvanic Current: Direct, continuous, unidirectional electric current.

Genes: Elements of the chromosomes by which hereditary characters are transmitted and determined.

Globular: Shaped like a globe or ball; popping out.

Glucides: Carbohydrates or juices (gastric juice). Most sweet substances are glucides.

Glycocoll: One of the amino acids found in numerous proteins.

Hormones: A substance secreted by a gland, acting upon some organ or tissue after having been carried through the blood vessels.

Hydrogen: A flammable, colorless, odorless, gaseous chemical element. The lightest of all known substances.

Hydrophobic: Cannot be diluted in water. Not capable of absorbing water.

Hydroscopic (Hydrophilic): Can be diluted in water. Capable of mixing with or absorbing water.

Hypolipoidic: Lacking fat. Synonym: alipoidic.

Intensity: The amount of force or energy produced by an electric current per time unit.

Introvert: A person whose interest is more in himself than in his environment or in other people.

Invaginated: That which folds itself inward.

Iodate: Iodic acid salt. Used as an antiseptic.

Ions: An electrically charged atom or group of atoms.

Iron: A mineral salt that activates the formation of the red blood cells.

Kaolin: A fine white, crumbly clay. Easily reduced to powder form.

Keratin: A tough, fibrous, insoluble protein, forming the principal matter of hair, nails, horn, and so forth.

Lipids: Fats and other substances with similar properties. Insoluble in water. Soluble in fat solvents and alcohol; greasy to the touch. Important constituents of living cells.

Liposoluble: Any substance soluble in fat solvents and alcohol.

Lubricating: A substance that reduces friction and ensures an oily protection.

Lysing: Tending to divide, split, digest, dissolve.

Magnesium: Antacid mineral salt. Certain skin diseases are the result of the lack of magnesium in the system.

Mandrel: A fine metal rod.

Melanin: A brownish-black pigment found in skin, hair, and other animal tissues.

Metaplasia: Conversion of one tissue into another, as of cartilage into bone.

Milium Nodule (Milia): An accumulation of sebum beneath the surface of the skin, resulting in a small whitish pimple (whitehead) .

Milliammeter: A device attached to an apparatus to measure the strength of an electric current; divided into units of one thousandth of an ampere.

Mucilage: Thick, sticky, viscous solution, produced in certain plants.

Multicellular: Consisting of many cells.

Neutral: That which is neither acidic nor basic. The intermediate state between acidity and alkalinity.

Neutron: One of the elementary particles found in the nucleus of most atoms. It is electrically uncharged.

Nevi, Neavi, Nevus: A colored spot on the skin. Usually congenital.

Nodules: Small knot or irregular rounded lump, protruding from the surface of the skin.

Nucleus: The central part of an atom.

Oestrogene (Estrogen): Female hormone.

Organic Acids: Acids found in the body, which dissolve and help eliminate urine, thus activating nutrition.

Osmosis: The tendency of a solution to pass through a semipermeable membrane, such as the walls of a living cell, into a solution of higher concentration, so as to equalize concentrations on both sides of the membrane.

Ostia: Plural for *ostium*. Orifice or opening of the pilosebaceous canal.

Oxygenating: To free of impurities. To assist respiration or breathing by supplementing oxygen.

Ozone: An unstable, pale blue gas with a penetrating odor. It is formed usually by a silent electrical discharge in the air. It has bactericidal and antiseptic properties.

Papillae: Plural for *papilla*. Any small nipplelike projection of connective tissue.

Papule: A small, usually inflammatory elevation of the skin; pimple.

Pectin: Organic substance found in the cellular membranes of certain plants.

Phenol: Disinfectant. Also used in the manufacture of certain pigments.

Phosphates: Mineral salts, one of the constituents of the principal organs.

Placental Extracts: Related to placenta, a vascular organ serving as nourishment for the fetus. Rich in vitamins, mineral salts, oligoelements, and so forth.

Plasma: The fluid part of the blood or lymph, which contains the cells.

Polyhedral: That which has more than six sides.

Potassium: A component of several mineral salts. One of the essential constituents of flesh and muscle.

Protein (Protide): Large molecule made of many subunits of amino acids, held together by peptide bonds. Proteins are found in all living tissues, such as skin, hair, nails.

Proteolytic: Organic substance that breaks down proteins to form simpler substances.

Proton: An elementary particle found in the nucleus of all atoms, which carries a positive electrical charge.

Pruritis (Pruritus): Intense itching of the skin without eruption.

Puberty: The period of time when one changes from childhood to adolescence. The state of physical development when sexual reproduction first becomes possible.

Pustule: A small elevation of the skin containing pus.

Regenerating: That which renews, restores, or helps to reconstruct tissue or part of a tissue.

Relieves Congestion: Activates circulation in blood vessels.

Reservoir: A receptacle or part of an apparatus that holds a fluid (water).

Resin: Viscous, organic substance exuded from various plants and trees.

Royal Jelly: Daily nutritive element of the queen bee. Highly nutritious mixture secreted by the maxillary glands in the young honey bee workers.

Saponification: The conversion of fats into soap.

Saponin: Any of a group of glucides of the same nature as soap.

Sauna: Vapor bath.

Scleroprotein: Any of a class of water-insoluble, fibrous animal proteins, including the keratins and collagens.

Sebum: The semiliquid, greasy secretion of the sebaceous glands.

Sedative Effect: Tending to soothe, calm.

Serum: Concentrated product, containing active ingredients in their pure state and sealed in sterile ampules.

Shock: An abrupt, sudden stimulation of the nerves, muscles, and so forth, accompanying the passage of electric current through the body.

Soluble: That which can be dissolved.

Soothing: Comforting, appeasing, calming, as by gentle treatment, such as relieving the pain of inflammation.

Spindle: The spindle-shaped bundle of nuclear fibers, which follow the chromosomes during one stage of mitosis.

Spontex: Pockets of sponge tissue used to insert the aluminium plates with the galvanic apparatus.

Starch (Glucide): Tasteless, odorless food substance found in many vegetable foods, such as potatoes, rice, corn.

Sterilized: That which has been freed from all living microorganisms by subjecting it to high temperatures or chemicals.

Synthesis: The artificial formation of a complex compound by combining its own elements.

Talc: A soft, usually massive and foliated mineral, magnesium silicate. Used to make talcum powder, and so forth.

Tannin: A mineral salt that has cicatrizant and astringent properties.

Thymol: Colorless, aromatic, crystalline compound, extracted from the volatile oil of thyme. Also used as an antiseptic.

Tonic: Producing or tending to produce good muscular tone or tension.

Vascularized: Containing many blood vessels.

Vasoconstrictor: Causing constriction of the blood vessels.

Vasodilator: Causing dilation of the blood vessels.

Ventouses (Suction Cups): Cupping glass; small glass cups used for suction.

Vertebrates: Having a backbone or spinal column.

Vitamin: An organic substance that is indispensable for the nutrition and balance of the organism.

Vitiligo: A disorder in which there is a loss of pigment, resulting in white patches of skin.

Wart: A small, usually hard tumorous growth on the skin, caused by a virus.

Water Soluble: Any substance that can be dissolved in water.

Yeast: Ferment, enzyme.

Bibliography

English Titles

"Better-Than-Ever Caring For Skin," *Vogue,* 167 (1977), 294–95.

"Black Woman's Guide To Skin Care," *McCalls,* 104 (1977), 140–41.

Bloom and Fawcett, *A Textbook of Histology.* Philadelphia: W. B. Saunders Company, 1970.

"Can Vitamins Help Your Skin?" *Vogue,* 165 (1975), 92.

Champion, R. H. and others, *An Introduction to the Biology of the Skin.* Philadelphia: J. B. Lippincott Company, 1970.

Chase, Deborah, *The Medically Based No-Nonsense Beauty Book.* New York: Alfred A. Knopf, Inc., 1974.

Culpeper, Nicholas, *The Complete Herbal.* Birmingham: Printed privately at the Kynoch Press.

"Diet That's Good for Your Skin," *Mademoiselle,* 82 (1976), 127–28.

"Environment Factor: Beauty/Health Hazard or Helper?" *Vogue,* 167 (1977), 164–67.

"How To Clean and Care For Your Skin, Interviews with Three Dermatologists," *Mademoiselle,* 83 (1977), 174–77.

Hyde, Margaret O., *Your Skin.* New York: McGraw-Hill Book Company, 1970.

Journal of Pharmaceutical Sciences, vol. 64 (June 1975.)

Lansing, Albert J., *Problems of Aging* (3rd ed.), Baltimore, Md.: The Williams & Wilkins Company.

Montagna, William, and P. F. Parakkal, *The Structure and Function of the Skin* (3rd ed.), New York: Academic Press, Inc., 1974.

"Nerves and Your Skin," *Harper's Bazaar,* 110 (1977), 126.

Penney, A., "Let's Face It," *New York Times Magazine,* December 18, 1977.

"Salon Facials: Where to Go," *Seventeen,* 36 (1977), 80–81.

Sauer, Gordon C., *Manual of Skin Diseases* (3rd ed.), Philadelphia: J. B. Lippincott Company, 1973.

Schoen, Linda A., ed., *The AMA Book of Skin and Hair Care.* Philadelphia: J. B. Lippincott Company, 1976.

"Scientific Skin Care," *Harper's Bazaar,* 110 (1977), 190–91.

Shelmire, J. Bedford, *The Art of Being Beautiful.* New York: St. Martin's Press, 1975.

Sternberg, Thomas Hunter, *More Than Skin Deep.* New York: Doubleday & Co., Inc., 1970.

"Unblemished Advice On Skin Care," *Today's Health,* 53 (1975), 36–39.

"Understanding Skin Care," *Family Health,* 9 (1977), 28–29.

Winter, Ruth, *A Consumer's Dictionary of Cosmetic Ingredients.* New York: Crown Publishers, Inc.

"What a Man Needs to Know About Skin Care," *Vogue,* 166 (1976), 212–13.

"Your Skin Checkup: Questions and Answers," *Redbook,* 143 (1974), 104–7.

Zizmor, Jonathan, and John Foreman, *Dr. Zizmor's Skin Care Book.* New York: Holt, Rinehart and Winston, 1977.

———, *Super Skin: The Doctor's Guide to a Beautiful Healthy Complexion.* New York: Thomas Y. Crowell Company, 1976.

French Titles

Adler, Irving, *L'Univers de l'Atôme.* Marabout Université.

Blum, Paul, "La Peau," *Que Sais-Je?* no. 558, P.U.F. (1966).

Bourgeois, Charles, "Chimie de la Beauté," *Que Sais-Je?* no. 901, P.U.F.

Bresse, Georges, *Morphologie et Physiologie Animales.* Paris: Librairie Larousse, 1968.

Chauchard, Paul, "Les Muscles," *Que Sais-Je?* no. 181, P.U.F. (1971).

Dictionnaire Encyclopédique Universel. Quillet and Grolier.

Dony, Gui, *Cours de Physio-Esthétique.* Brussels: Electricité–Actinologie, 1966.

Dumoulin, J., and G. de Bessihop, *Electrothérapie.* Librarie Maloine, 1966.

Duval, Clement, "L'Oxygène," *Que Sais-Je?* no. 1273, P.U.F. (1967).

Firket, Henri, "La Cellule Vivante," *Que Sais-Je?* no. 989, P.U.F. (1969).

Gallot, Suzanne, "Les Vitamines," *Que Sais-Je?* no. 12, P.U.F. (1972).

Graciansky, Pierre de, "La Dermatologie," *Que Sais-Je?* no. 1132, P.U.F. (1969).

Guillerme, Jacques, "L'Ultraviolet," *Que Sais-Je?* no. 662, P.U.F. (1974).

Hadni, Armand, "L'Infrarouge," *Que Sais-Je?* no. 497, P.U.F. (1975).

Halpern, Bernard, "L'Allergie," *Que Sais-Je?* no. 1201, P.U.F. (1969).

Messier, Bernard, *Histologie Générale,* Département d'Anatomie, Faculté de Médecine. La Librairie de l'Université de Montréal, 1972–1973.

Messier, Paul Emil, *Introduction à l'Ultrastructure Cellulaire.* Les Presses de l'Université de Montréal, 1971.

Morand, Genevieve, "Matière, Electricité, Energie," *Que Sais-Je?* no. 291, P.U.F. (1973).

Nourse, Alan E., "Le Corps," *Le Monde des Sciences,* Collection Life, 1968.

Nouvelle Encyclopédie Pratique d'Electricité. vol. 1, no. 11, Librairie Aristide.

Pfeiffer, John, *La Cellule.* R. Laffont Sciences, 1969.

Prettre, Marcel, "Catalyse et Catalyseurs," *Que Sais-Je?* no. 240, P.U.F. (1970).

Relyveld, Edgar, and Jean Claude Cherman, "Les Protéines," *Que Sais-Je?* no. 679, P.U.F. (1970).

Rey, Pierre, "Les Hormones," *Que Sais-Je?* no. 39, P.U.F.

Rocchiccioli-Deltcheff, C., "Le pH et sa Mesure," *Que Sais-Je?* no. 1248, P.U.F. (1970).

Stolkowski, Joseph, "Les Enzymes," *Que Sais-Je?* no. 434, P.U.F. (1973).

Index

D

E

H

I

L

O

P

T

U

V

W

Z

BALANCED NUTRITION FOR A HEALTHY SKIN

	Natural Sources	Effects on the Skin
VITAMIN A (B carotene or retinol)	Milk, cheese, spinach, broccoli, lettuce, asparagus, carrots, squash, sweet potatoes, tomatoes, cantaloupes, peaches, apricots, watermelon, liver.	Prevents desquamation (peeling), scabs, and strias.
VITAMIN B_1 (thiamin)	Milk, almonds, peanuts, wheat cereals, oatmeal, rice, salmon, oysters, mackerel, pork, ham, beef heart.	Offers an important contribution to the numerous intercellular reactions. The secretion of Vitamin B_1 through the skin is believed to be a good insect repellent.
VITAMIN B_2 (riboflavin)	Milk, yogurt, ice cream, broccoli, spinach, enriched cereals, oatmeal, liver, kidney, beef heart.	Helps oxygenation and prevents desquamation.
VITAMIN B_5 (pantothenic acid)	Yeast, enriched cereals, soy beans, liver, egg yolk.	Helps prevent hair falling, alopecia areata (hair falling in patches), and hair greying.
VITAMIN B_6 (pyridoxine)	Milk, oranges, pears, bananas, yeast, cereals, oatmeal, liver.	Very important to the skin and nervous system. Helps prevent dermatosis scaling (psoriasis) and seborrhaeic scaling (scabs).
VITAMIN C (ascorbic acid)	Oranges, grapefruits, lemons, limes, strawberries, raspberries, mulberries, cantaloupes, watermelon, Brussels sprouts, cauliflower, cabbage, broccoli, green peppers, tomatoes, watercress, turnips.	Facilitates healing of scars. Helps prevent scurvy. Provides nutritive elements to the melanin.

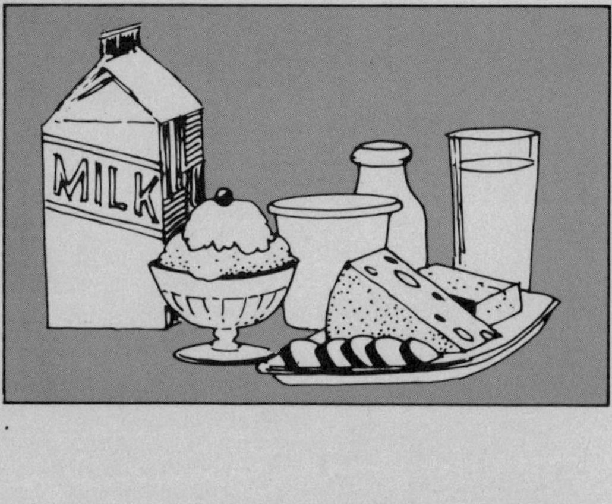

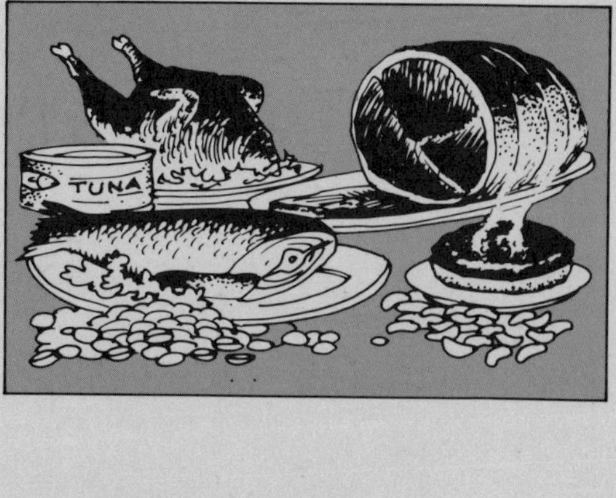